USE OF BOTULINUM TOXIN TYPE A
IN PAIN MANAGEMENT

USE OF BOTULINUM TOXIN TYPE A IN PAIN MANAGEMENT

A Clinician's Guide
2nd edition

EDITOR

MARTIN K. CHILDERS, DO
Associate Professor
Department of Physical Medicine and Rehabilitation
University of Missouri–Columbia
Columbia, Missouri

CONTRIBUTING AUTHORS

K. Roger Aoki, PhD
Vice President, Neurotoxin Research
Allergan, Inc.
Irvine, California

Yuemei G. Corliss, PhD
Allergan, Inc.
Irvine, California

Patrick J. Hogan III, DO
Director, Puget Sound Neurology
Headache & Movement Disorder Clinic
Tacoma, Washington

Eric G. Kassel, PharmD
Director, Regional Scientific Services
Allergan, Inc.
Irvine, California

Divakara Kedlaya, MD
Assistant Professor
Department of Physical Medicine and Rehabilitation
Center for Pain Management and Research
Loma Linda University Medical Center
Loma Linda, California

David G. Simons, MD
Retired
Covington, Georgia

Diane Simison, PhD
Principal, Epinomics Research, Inc.
Alexandria, Virginia

Daniel J. Wilson, PhD
Assistant Professor
Southwest Missouri State University
Springfield, Missouri

Prescribing information, dosing, side effects and adverse reactions described in this book may change. The reader should carefully review package insert information prior to prescribing any of the medications referenced.

To purchase additional copies of this book call 1 (573) 474-8161, Fax: 1 (573) 474-6763, or email: aiscolmo@aol.com

ISBN 0-9663-422-9-1
Library of Congress Control Number: 2002102532

Printed in the United States of America

Illustration 4.1 created by and reproduced with permission of Patrick J. Hogan III.

Illustrations 7.12 (inset), 7.13 (inset), 7.17, 7.18 created by and reproduced with permission of Kari C. Childers.

Illustrations 4.2–4.4, 5.1, 5.3–5.5, 7.1–7.16, 7.19–7.21 reproduced with permission from Wolf-Heidegger's Atlas of Human Anatomy, edited by Petra Kopf-Maier, S. Karger AG, Basel, 2001.

CONTENTS

TREATMENT OF PAINFUL SYNDROMES OF MUSCLE REMAINS INCOMPLETELY understood and controversial. While the use of botulinum toxin type A (BTX-A) in the treatment of conditions associated with involuntary muscle contraction, such as focal dystonia and spasticity, is supported by prospective, randomized clinical research, comparable research in pain syndromes remains to be fully explored. Accordingly, therapy with BTX-A for such "off-label" use should be carefully considered. The purpose of this introductory guide is to provide both general direction and practical details for the busy clinician. The anatomic drawings for injection localization and accompanying dosing information are intended only as general guidelines—therapy with BTX-A must always be individualized, not only for the patient's needs but also for the clinician's expertise. This handbook should be used as a convenient reference source and not as a substitute for clinical training in the use of botulinum toxin.

Martin K. Childers, D.O.

USE OF BOTULINUM TOXIN TYPE A IN PAIN MANAGEMENT

INTRODUCTION

Martin K. Childers

THIS HANDBOOK OUTLINES USES OF BOTULINUM TOXIN TYPE A (BTX-A; Botox, Allergan, Inc.) for pain management. Although the United States Food and Drug Administration (FDA) licensed uses for BTX-A address pain management for cervical dystonia only, this product is used by a range of medical specialists to address pain control of various etiologies (Jankovic and Brin, 1991). However, there is insufficient available information to directly address clinical guidelines or provide the necessary knowledge to most appropriately use BTX-A for pain management. The purpose of this handbook, therefore, is to provide some clinical guidance to physicians regarding the use of BTX-A, based upon similar applications in a variety of neuromuscular disorders.

The text highlights essential features one should know about BTX-A before treating patients for pain, and additional sources of information are listed at the end of the text in the Appendix.

TOPICS

- Pharmacology and pain
- Concept of LD_{50}
- Dosing and administration
- Injection methods

- Treatment(s) which might be helpful in conjunction with BTX-A therapy
- Contraindications

APPLICATIONS

In 2001, the FDA licensed BTX-A in the United States for treatment of the following in patients over the age of 12 years:

- strabismus—a condition in which one or both eyes do not move together in tandem
- essential blepharospasm—involuntary blinking
- hemifacial spasm—involuntary facial muscle spasms
- cervical dystonia and pain related to cervical dystonia

But in addition to the approved uses in the United States, there are other published uses of BTX-A, which include:

achalasia	hyperhydrosis
anismus	myofascial pain syndrome
cervical dystonia	occupational dystonia
detrusor-sphincter	pain (muscle spasm)
dysinergia	headache
essential blepharospasm	piriformis muscle syndrome
essential tremor	spasmotic dysphonia
facial wrinkles	spasticity
hemifacial spasm	strabismus

In addition to publications, noteworthy medical organizations have commented on the effectiveness and safety of BTX-A. The National Institutes of Health Consensus Development Conference published a statement in 1990 summarizing indications and contraindications of BTX-A usage for the treatment of a variety of conditions (National Institutes of Health, 1991). The NIH conference endorsed the use of BTX-A as safe and effective for the symptomatic treatment of adductor spasmodic dysphonia, blepharospasm, cervical dystonia, hemifacial spasm, jaw-closing oromandibular dystonia, and strabismus. The same year, the Therapeutics and Technology Assessment Subcommittee of the American Academy of Neurology further endorsed the use of BTX-A for the symptomatic treatment of these conditions (American Academy of Neurology, 1994).

EMG CONSIDERATIONS

The use of electromyography (EMG) for injection localization of BTX-A in pain management can be helpful and at times improve clinical response. However, previous experience with EMG is not necessary, since its use for injection localization is much simpler than for diagnostic purposes. EMG does require a working knowledge of functional anatomy and neuromuscular physiology (Gnatz, 2001). Relevant information is offered throughout this text and the topic is examined in some detail in Chapter 7 for readers not familiar with this tool.

REFERENCES

American Academy of Neurology. Training guidelines for the use of botulinum toxin for the treatment of neurologic disorders. Report of the Therapeutics and Technology Assessment Subcommittee of the American Academy of Neurology. *Neurology* 44:2401–2403, 1994.

Gnatz S: *EMG Basics.* AIS Publishing, Columbia MO, 2001.

Jankovic J, Brin MF. Therapeutic uses of botulinum toxin. [Review]. *N Engl J Med* 324:1186–1194, 1991.

National Institutes of Health. Consensus conference. Clinical uses of botulinum toxin. National Institutes of Health. [Review]. *Conn Med* 55:471–477, 1991.

CHAPTER ONE

Eric G. Kassel

Divakara Kedlaya

OVERVIEW OF CLINICAL USE

THIS CHAPTER BRIEFLY SUMMARIZES THERAPEUTIC USES OF BOTULINUM TOXIN across the clinical spectrum. Because painful conditions exist in many settings, clinicians should be aware of other circumstances that might be amenable to treatment with the neurotoxin. This chapter summarizes botulinum toxin use in a range of disorders.

FOCAL DYSTONIAS

Cervical Dystonia

Botulinum toxin type A (BTX-A) has been clinically used for the treatment of cervical dystonia (spasmodic torticollis) since the early 1980s. It was approved by the U.S. Food and Drug Administration (FDA) in 1989 under the brand name Botox (Allergan, Inc.) for the treatment of blepharospasm, strabismus, and seventh cranial nerve disorders in children 12 years of age and older. In December 2000 BTX-A, Botox was approved for the treatment of cervical dystonia in adults to decrease the severity of abnormal head position and neck pain associated with cervical dystonia. In a phase 3 randomized, double-blind, placebo-controlled trial, 170 cervical dystonia patients who responded to previous treatments with Botox were randomized to receive Botox as in prior, open-label treatments or placebo. The active treatment group showed significant improvement in their Cervical Dystonia Severity Scale, Physician Global Assessment Scale, as well as improvement in pain scores. The average dose received was 236 U (198–300 U) lasting 3 months (Botox prescribing information, Allergan, Inc.). Long-term safety and efficacy has been established with a small incidence of dry mouth and dysphagia with a historical secondary nonresponsiveness of approximately 5% (Kessler et al, 1999). Furthermore, BTX-A improved functional impairment, disability, pain, handicap, and quality of life in patients with cervical dystonia (Brans et al, 1998; Lu et al, 1995).

Botulinum toxin type B (BTX-B) is only the second serotype of botulinum toxin that has entered the U.S. commercial market since the concept of botulinum toxins as a clinically useful treatment was developed in the late 1960s. BTX-B was approved in late 2000 under the brand name Myobloc (Elan Pharmaceuticals) for the treatment of patients with cervical dystonia to reduce the severity of abnormal head position and neck pain associated with cervical dystonia. BTX-B efficacy was evaluated in two phase 3, randomized, double-blind, placebo-controlled trials of adults with cervical dystonia who were perceived to be responding to BTX-A previously. In the first study, 109 patients received placebo, 5000 U, or 10,000 U of Myobloc and in the second study 77 patients received either placebo or 10,000 U of Myobloc. Subjects underwent a single treatment session by investigators who selected two to four muscles involved in the patient's cervical dystonia. There was a significant improvement in Toronto Western Spasmodic Torticollis Rating Scale (TWSTRS) total, Patient Global, and Physician Global scores for both the 5000 U and 10,000 U groups with no statistically significant difference between the two treatment groups. TWSTRS subscales of Severity, Pain, and Disability were all significant in the 10,000 U treatment group with pain the only significant improvement in the 5000 U treatment arms. Analysis of the first controlled trial showed a return to baseline status between weeks 12 and 16. The most common side effects occurring in the two studies were dry mouth, dysphagia, dyspepsia, and injection site pain. Dry mouth and dysphagia occurred in 34% and 25%, respectively, of patients in the 10,000 U group, and in 12% and 10% of patients in the

5000 U group, compared with 3% in the placebo groups. Rates of neutralizing antibody formation were 10% at 1 year and 18% at 18 months; the effect of the neutralizing antibodies was not evaluated (Brashear et al, 1999, Brin et al, 1999). Practical aspects of the use of BTX-A for cervical dystonia is described by Kedlaya et al, 1999.

Blepharospasm

Blepharospasm, or eyelid closure, is an involuntary spasmodic contraction of the orbicularis oculi muscle of unknown origin. Blepharospasm is one of the original three label indications for the use of Botox (BTX-A) neurotoxin complex. It involves increased frequency and force of eye closure, often progresses rapidly, and frequently results in functional blindness. In an open label study, 27 patients received injections of BTX-A as Botox in six sites on each side, each containing 2.0 U. All patients had failed conventional oral drug therapy. Twenty-five patients reported improvement within 48 hours, one patient was controlled with a higher dosage at 13 weeks, and the last patient reported mild improvement but remained functionally impaired (Arthurs et al, 1987).

In a double-blind, placebo-controlled study, eight patients receiving BTX-A, Botox significantly improved compared with the placebo group. The effects lasted an average of 12.5 weeks. In blepharospasm patients, 90–98% reported moderate to excellent improvement in spasm intensity and significant improvement in disability while experiencing infrequent side effects, mainly ptosis and facial weakness, when treated with BTX-A (Chang et al, 1999, Thussu et al, 1999). A double-blind crossover trial in 212 patients compared two different commercially available BTX-A products, Botox and Dysport. No difference was found in duration, but ptosis occurred significantly less in the Botox group than in the Dysport group at a 1:4 Botox:Dysport dosage ratio (Price et al, 1997).

Laryngeal Dystonias

Laryngeal dystonia, or spasmodic dysphonia, is a focal neurological disorder characterized by action-induced spasms of the vocal cords. Adductor-type spasmodic dysphonia is the most common presentation, and is characterized by a strained, harsh voice with tremor, breaks, breathiness, and inappropriate pitch. Abductor type is far less common and is characterized by a breathy, effortful voice with abrupt termination causing whispered segments of speech.

In a retrospective analysis of more than 900 patients with adductor and abductor laryngeal dystonia over a 12-year period, 87% had adductor-type spasmodic dysphonia and 13% presented with abductor type. In adductor type, 3.096 ± 3.1 U (0.005–30 U) produced an approximately 90% return of normal function lasting a little over 15 weeks. In abductor-type spasmodic dysphonia, 2.163 ± 1.07 U (0.5–6.25 U) produced an approximate 67% return of normal function lasting over 10 weeks (Blitzer et al, 1998; Gibbs and Blitzer, 2000). Unilateral injections seem to decrease the incidence of side effects, mainly dysphagia, when compared with the bilateral technique (Langeveld et al, 1998). The most common side effects occurring from dysphonia injections are spasms, hoarseness, breathiness, and dysphagia. They resolve in 4–6 weeks, whereas voice improvement lasts 12–15 weeks (Liu et al, 1998).

Limb Dystonia

Focal dystonia of the hand (writer's cramp) is characterized by muscle spasms that cause difficulties in fine hand motor control (Cohen et al, 1989). This subset of dystonia can be fixed or task-specific, and is often disabling and poorly responsive to medical therapy (Yoshimura et al, 1992). Since the early 1990s, botulinum toxin therapy has been used in the treatment of hand dystonia such as writer's cramp.

In double-blind fashion, 10 patients received BTX-A for writer's cramp. There was significant improvement in subjective rating, objective testing, and physicians' rating of performance (Cole et al, 1995). An additional 20 patients with writer's cramp were studied in a double-blind, placebo-controlled, crossover fashion. Patient improvement was measured objectively by observed pain control at 0, 2, and 6 weeks. Twelve patients had improvement of pain control after BTX-A injection with four having significant improvement (Tsui et al, 1993). Long-term botulinum toxin treatment was assessed in focal hand dystonia in an open-label fashion. Fifty-three patients were followed for up to 6 years. Eighty-one percent of patients improved with at least one injection session, with 65% of the injections producing transient weakness. The dose of toxin fluctuated within a range of 20 U with side effects being mild and transient. Botulinum toxin therapy was considered safe and effective for long-term management of focal hand dystonia (Karp et al, 1994).

Oromandibular Dystonia

Oromandibular dystonia is a collective group of neurological disorders that involve the temporomandibular joint, masticatory muscles, and associated structures. Traditional therapy for many patients is not totally effective and often fails to relieve the pain resulting from the syndrome.

Freund and Schwartz (1998) studied 19 patients referred to their surgery clinic for temporomandibular disorder (TMD). The patients received a total dose of 25 or 50 U BTX-A. Two of the eight patients in the low-dose group reported improvement, whereas 10 of 11 patients in the high-dose group reported decreased pain and general improvement. The only notable side effects were weakness while chewing, which correlated with general improvement. In a retrospective assessment of 162 patients treated with botulinum toxin for oromandibular dystonia over 10 years, the average dose used in the masseters was 54.2 U, 28.6 U in the submentalis complex, with an average duration of 16.4 weeks. The mean global effect was 3.1 out of 4, with 4 being complete relief of the dystonia (Tan and Jankovic, 1999).

Truncal Dystonia

Truncal dystonia is manifested by involuntary back arching. It is often associated with severe pain and disability, and rarely responds to pharmacological intervention.

In one report, five patients with severe idiopathic or tardive truncal and cervical dystonia were treated with BTX-A (Botox) injections into the paravertebral muscles of the lumbar region in four to six sites. Each site was injected with 25–50 U of BTX-A with a mean dose of 210 U (150–300 U). By blinded videotape evaluation, objective improvement was found in three patients with a mean truncal dystonia score improving by 37% and movement range improvement of 20–80% (mean, 46%). All patients who experienced pain reported substantial improvement, no worsening of dystonia, and no adverse events. The authors concluded that botulinum toxin injections offered a potent new treatment for truncal dystonia (Comella et al, 1998).

SPASTICITY

Stroke

Spasticity following stroke presents numerous problems, including increased muscle tone, abnormal limb posture, increased activity of antagonist muscles, and hyperactive cutaneous and tendon reflexes. The prevalence of disability in stroke survivors is high, and the management of spasticity following stroke requires establishing realistic goals with a combination of treatment modalities to produce the best outcomes (O'Brien et al, 1996).

In post-stroke upper limb spasticity, double-blind, placebo-controlled trials demonstrated that reduction in spasticity after BTX-A injections resulted in a significant decrease in disability and caretaker burden (Bakheit et al, 2001; Bhakta et al, 1996, 2000; Simpson et al, 1996; Smith et al, 2000). In 39 patients with chronic upper limb spasticity, participants received intramuscular injections of either placebo, 75, 150, or 300 U of BTX-A (Botox). Following injections, significant improvements ensued in the Ashworth Scale, as well as physician and patient Global Assessment of Response to Treatment Scales (Simpson et al, 1996). Similarly, 40 patients with spasticity in a functionally useless arm were randomized to either placebo or a total dose of 1000 MU of BTX-A (Dysport) divided between the elbow, wrist, and finger flexors. After treatment, there were significant improvements in the modified Ashworth scores, muscle power scores, joint movement measures, and pain scores. Disability and caretaker burden improved significantly as well. The authors concluded that BTX-A is useful in treating patients with stroke who have self-care difficulties due to arm spasticity and that caretaker burden should also be considered when making treatment decisions (Bhakta et al, 2000).

In a recently presented abstract, 126 patients with post-stroke spasticity were randomized to receive 200–240 U of BTX-A (Botox) or placebo in the wrist and finger flexors. At baseline, all patients demonstrated an Ashworth score of 3 or higher (out of 4). The Ashworth score, Physician and Patient Global Assessment score, and the Disability Assessment Scale (DAS) were significantly improved at 1, 4, 6, 8, and 12 weeks after injection. (The DAS is a four-point scale grading the effect of spasticity on four domains of hygiene, dressing, pain, and limb position.) Improvement in the DAS correlated with the changes in the Ashworth scores, as well as the Physician and Patient Global Assessment scales (Brashear et al, 2001).

Traumatic Brain Injury

The paucity of information on the treatment of spasticity in the patient with traumatic brain injury does not correlate well with clinical practice. Much of the literature for general spasticity has been extrapolated to current clinical practice.

Effects of botulinum toxin were studied in 21 patients with traumatic brain injury who had distal upper limb spasticity of the wrist and finger flexors. Patients were given 20 to 40 U of BTX-A per muscle, administered under electromyographic (EMG) guidance. The patient's range of motion and modified Ashworth Scale were assessed at 2 to 4 weeks post injection. After injection, significant improvements from baseline were noted in range of motion measures and mean modified Ashworth scores in all patients (Yablon et al, 1996). Another similar study has also shown the efficacy of BTX-A in spasticity due to traumatic brain injury (Pavesi et al, 1998).

Cerebral Palsy

Cerebral palsy (CP) is a syndrome caused by central nervous system damage that appears early in life and is characterized by erratic control of movement and posture. Symptoms can be due to loss of selective motor control, abnormal muscle tone, imbalance between agonist/antagonist muscles, and/or impaired balance. The goal of therapy is to maximize function and minimize joint contracture and other secondary problems. Botulinum toxin therapy has become a standard practice in the treatment of patients with CP who are hypertonic and whose abnormal tone interferes with function, and in those patients who are likely to develop joint contractures due to the abnormal tone (Russman et al, 1997).

In a randomized, controlled, single-blinded trial, 29 patients with upper limb spasticity due to CP were either injected with BTX-A (Botox) in the biceps, forearm, and adductor pollicus and received occupational therapy, or received occupational therapy alone. Outcomes were evaluated at 0, 1, 3, and 6 months using Ashworth scores, Quality of Upper Extremity Skills Test (QUEST), goniometry measurements, and grip strength. There was significant improvement after treatment in the botulinum toxin group in some of these outcomes. These findings supported the idea that botulinum toxin therapy can improve upper extremity function in children with hemiplegia who have moderate spasticity (Fehlings et al, 2000).

In a similar randomized, double-blind study of 14 patients with upper limb hemiplegia due to CP, BTX-A therapy significantly increased maximum active elbow and thumb extension and significantly reduced tone at the wrist and elbow. The decrease in muscle tone was clinically apparent and the patients and parents perceived the change as beneficial (Corry et al, 1997). In 54 subjects with CP, paraparesis with lower limb spasticity was the most common clinical finding. BTX-A (Botox) treatment was tailored depending on the child's age and degree of spasticity. Initial dose per session was 6–8 U/kg with subsequent sessions of 8–10 U/kg. Subsequently, there was a significant decrease in spasticity in 92% of patients as noted by a 2+ or more decrease in the Ashworth Scale. Gait also improved in 80% of subjects, while muscle spasms improved in 5 of 5 and pain improved in 7 of 10 subjects. Parents observed improvement in their children's sleep (5/6), hygiene (7/9), ease of dressing (4/5), and irritability (9/11). In several children, corrective orthopedic surgery was delayed to an older age when surgical results might be more predictable (Jabbari et al, 1998).

In 114 patients with CP and equinus positioning of the foot during stance, either BTX-A (Botox) 4 U/kg or placebo was injected into the medial and lateral gastrocnemius of each involved leg. There was subsequent significant improvement in the Composite Physician Rating Scale scores, ankle range of motion measures, and gait evaluations in patients treated with botulinum toxin (Koman et al, 2000).

Multiple Sclerosis

Multiple sclerosis (MS) is an inflammatory disease of the central nervous system and a major cause of neurologic disability in young and middle-aged adults. Characteristic cerebral plaques can affect numerous areas and cause neurologic symptoms that accrue over time. Symptoms include pain, paresthesias, weakness, ataxia, fatigue, tremors, increased muscle tone, and spasticity.

BTX-A was evaluated for the treatment of adductor spasticity secondary to MS in a blinded, placebo-controlled fashion in 74 patients. Patients received 0, 500, 1000, or 1500 U of BTX-A (Dysport) and were evaluated over 12 weeks. Muscle tone and pain were reduced in all groups. Although a dose–response effect was not statistically significant, there appeared to be a trend toward efficacy and duration of effect with higher doses. Side effects were significantly higher in the higher-dose group. The authors concluded that an optimal dose of 500–1000 U of BTX-A (Dysport) divided between legs was effective in adductor spasticity due to MS (Hyman et al, 2000). This decrease in spasticity of MS origin has been documented with other formulations of BTX-A as well. BTX-A (Botox) was found to be beneficial in improving spasticity and pain of the upper and lower limbs secondary to MS, and in acquired nystagmus and facial myokymia (Borg-Stein et al, 1993; Sedano et al, 2000).

NONDYSTONIC DISORDERS OF INVOLUNTARY MUSCLE ACTIVITY

Hemifacial Spasm

Hemifacial spasm (HFS) is a peripherally induced, involuntary, unilateral, irregular, tonic or clonic contraction of the muscles innervated by the ipsilateral facial nerve (Wang and Jankovic, 1998). HFS is a disorder with an undesirable effect on lifestyle and social activities and can be treated medically, surgically, or with botulinum toxin therapy. BTX-A has become the mainstay of therapy for HFS in the last decade.

In a study of 58 patients with HFS, 86.2% had excellent improvement in a spasm intensity scale while 6.8% had moderate improvement. Complications included mild facial weakness, ptosis, swelling, and bruising (Chang et al, 1999). In a prospective descriptive study in which 175 patients were injected around the eye for HFS with BTX-A (Dysport), 158 were treated four times and, on the visual analogue scale, showed a response rate of 97% lasting 3–4 months. The most common side effect was ptosis (Jitpimolmard, 1998). In a prospective study of 250 patients with HFS receiving 30 U in four injection sites over the involved facial muscles, 81% of patients had excellent improvement, 10% moderate improvement, 8% mild improvement, and 2% did not respond. Complications included mild transient facial weakness and ptosis. The effects generally lasted 3–6 months. The authors concluded that BTX-A was a simple, safe, and effective treatment for HFS (Poungvarin and Viriyavejakul, 1992).

Tremors

Essential tremor is a common movement disorder that can cause disability leading to physical and emotional difficulties. Pharmacologic treatment options include anticonvulsants, antidepressants, antipsy-chotics, beta-blockers, and methylxanthine derivatives (Koller et al, 2000). Treatment with BTX-A has been evaluated in voice, hand, and head tremors.

Voice Tremors

In essential voice tremor, BTX-A was injected into the thyroarytoid, cricothyroid, and thyrohyoid muscles. The beneficial effects were seen with significant decreases in tremor during controlled speech, fre-quency variations, and vowel phonation. Success rates were reported at 50–65% (Hertegard et al, 2000). In a prospective, open-label, crossover study, 10 patients received 2.5 U of BTX-A (Botox) bilater-ally or 15 U unilaterally with crossover occurring after 16–18 weeks. The authors concluded that patients subjectively improved in vocal effort, even though objective findings were difficult to measure (Warrick et al, 2000).

Hand Tremors

In a randomized, double-blind, placebo-controlled study to evaluate BTX-A (Botox) therapy in hand tremor, 25 patients with 2+ to 4+ scores on the tremor severity scale received 50 U BTX-A or placebo in the wrist flexors and extensors of the dominant hand. If patients failed therapy, they became eligible to receive 100 U 4 weeks later. Four weeks post injection, 75% of patients treated with botulinum toxin and 27% of those who received placebo reported mild to moderate improvement in tremor. There was no significant improvement in func-tional ratings scales. Postural accelerometry measures showed 30% decrease in amplitude in 9/12 patients treated with botulinum toxin. Finger weakness was the only reported side effect (Jankovic et al, 1996).

In another randomized, double-blind, controlled study of 133 patients with essential hand tremor, BTX-A injections showed signif-icant improvement of postural, but not kinetic, hand tremors and rsult-ed in limited functional efficacy (Brin et al, 2001).

In an open-label study to determine the utility of botulinum toxin injections into the forearm and arm for severe hand tremor, 26 patients (12 with Parkinson's disease and 14 with essential tremor) were observed. Of this group, 17% of those with Parkinson's tremor and 21% of those with essential tremor experienced quantitative changes in tremor amplitude ($> 50\%$ decrease) compared with pretreatment measurements. Over 38% of patients reported moderate to marked subjective improvement 6 weeks after injection. The authors concluded that although objective improvement was difficult to measure, botulinum toxin injections improved tremor in some patients, especially those with essential hand tremor (Trosch and Pullman, 1994).

Head Tremors

Head tremor has been the object of botulinum toxin therapy for some time. Forty-three patients with head tremor presented for BTX-A (Dysport) injections. All patients were assessed with the Tsui Scale and quantitative recordings of head tremor with bidirectional accelerometer measurements. Muscle selection was based on visible and palpable tremors and on EMG analysis. Forty patients had significant improvement on the Tsui Scale, and pain scores decreased significantly (Wissel et al, 1997). In a double-blind, placebo-controlled study, 10 patients with essential head tremor received two treatments 3 months apart with BTX-A (Botox) or saline into the sternocleidomastoid and the splenius capitis muscles. There was significant subjective and objective improvement in five patients after BTX-A therapy. The authors concluded that BTX-A might be a useful treatment for essential head tremor (Pahwa et al, 1995).

Tics

Gilles de la Tourette syndrome (TS) is a complex movement disorder, which may present with multiple motor tics and vocalizations, a fluctuating but chronic course, and age of onset younger than 18 years (Trimble et al, 1998). Botulinum toxin therapy in the treatment of tics was reported, with the vocal tics of TS often targeted with laryngeal injections.

In an early pilot study to determine efficacy in the treatment of such tics, 10 male patients with TS with focal tics were studied. Five patients had blinking and blepharospasm rendering them "blind" and five patients had severe and painful dystonic tics involving neck muscles. All 10 patients experienced moderate to marked improvement after BTX-A treatment. Patients noted improvements in intensity and frequency of the tics as well as improvement in the premonitory urges that preceded the tics (Krauss and Jankovic, 1996).

Thirty-five patients with TS were treated with BTX-A (Botox) in the site of their most problematic tics. The mean duration of effect was 14.4 weeks with the mean dose per visit being 119.9 U. Over 76% reported marked improvement of symptoms. The tics decreased in frequency, duration, and intensity with total resolution in five patients, and 84% of patients had marked relief of their premonitory sensations. The authors concluded that BTX-A is an effective and well-tolerated treatment of TS-associated tics. Side effects were infrequent and self-limiting (Kwak et al, 2000).

In a similar study, 450 patients with TS were treated with baclofen, BTX-A (Botox), or both. In this study, 186 patients received botulinum toxin A; 35 patients reported complete control of their motor tics after botulinum toxin therapy, and less success in control of their vocal tics. Reinstitution of baclofen in 31 of those patients resulted in resolution of vocal tics. Four patients received injections in their vocal cords, which was followed by a 30% reduction in vocal tics. The authors concluded that BTX-A and baclofen could be useful in the treatment of TS in children (Awaad, 1999).

Myokymia and Synkinesis

Myokymia is an involuntary undulating, vermicular movement that spreads across facial muscles and is often seen in patients with MS, brain stem glioma, or stroke. Patients who experience these disorders may find relief with botulinum toxin therapy.

In two cases, patients with MS and continuous hemifacial myokymia lasting up to 1 month were treated with botulinum toxin therapy. One patient was treated for left facial myokymia with 2.5 U of BTX-A (Botox) in the upper and lower lids, cheek, and perioral muscles, much as in hemifacial spasm. The second patient was treated for left orbicular myokymia with 2.5 U in five points around the left eye. Both patients experienced complete relief of symptoms (Sedano et al, 2000). In a patient who experienced trismus associated with post-radiation myokymia and muscle spasm, 25 U of BTX-A (Botox) was injected into each masseter and mylohyoid muscle with EMG guidance. This patient noticed clinical improvement in 3 days that lasted 5 weeks (Lou et al, 1995).

Synkinesis refers to involuntary muscle contractions that follow a voluntary muscle contraction. A group of patients with facial nerve palsy who were experiencing facial spasm and synkinesis were injected with 2.5–5 U of BTX-A into the affected muscles. They reported good response without adverse effects, and it was concluded that botulinum toxin therapy within 6 weeks of onset of paralysis could be efficacious (Smet-Dielman et al, 1993).

Facial synkinesis and asymmetry are often a common outcome of facial nerve palsy. Twenty-four patients with synkinesis and asymmetry affecting the eye and mouth were injected with BTX-A. Sixty-eight of 72 treatments produced improved cosmesis. Dose-related complications were mild and transient, and there was no difference in efficacy of high doses compared with low doses (Armstrong et al, 1996).

Myoclonus

Myoclonus (tensor veli palatini muscle—middle ear—causing tinnitus) of the individual muscles in the head or neck can cause pain and distort speech and hearing. These symptoms can interfere with normal function and even prevent walking. Because of inadequate response or intolerable side effects, oral medications are often abandoned early in treatment.

In nine patients with segmental, generalized, and focal myoclonus, BTX-A (Botox) in doses of 4.9–45.4 U/kg was administered in the involved myoclonic musculature. EMG guidance was used in all cases, with marked overall improvement in the Global Assessment score in all cases. One patient experienced arm weakness and did not complete treatment. The ability of BTX-A to improve function with an absence of side effects at higher than usual doses warranted a closer look in the management of myoclonus resistant to conventional therapies (Awaad et al, 1999). In two cases of palatal myoclonus, 7.5 U of BTX-A (Botox) was injected into each tensor veli palatini muscle in one patient. One month later, the patient reported a decrease in clicking on the right, while clicking on the left had stopped; however, the patient complained of fullness on the same side that led to ventilation tube placement. The patient continued to receive botulinum toxin injections every 3–4 months thereafter.

In the second case, a patient with an 18-month history of bilateral tinnitus received 10 U of botulinum toxin into the left tensor veli palatini muscle. Two weeks later, only right-sided tinnitus remained. The patient subsequently received 10 U of BTX-A into the right tensor veli palatini muscle. Two days later tinnitus ceased. Upon return of symptoms 2 years later, the patient received 4 U BTX-A every 2 months on alternating sides, and thereafter remained symptom free (Bryce and Morrison, 1998). In another case report, a 59-year-old women with gradual onset of bilateral ear clicking received 5 U of BTX-A into the insertion of the tensor veli palatini and also into the insertion of the levator veli palatini muscle bilaterally. The patient reported resolution of ear clicking and palatal twitching after the first day and remained symptom free 7 months later (Varney et al, 1996).

Hereditary Muscle Cramps

Since botulinum toxin therapy is widely used in the treatment of hyperkinetic movement disorders, it is thought to have a role in the treatment of chronic muscle cramping syndromes. Five patients with benign cramp-fasciculation syndrome of autosomal dominant inheritance were treated with BTX-A (Dysport). All patients had a long history of disabling generalized muscular cramps predominantly affecting leg muscles. BTX-A was injected bilaterally with 350–400 U into the gastrocnemius muscles and 80–100 U into the small flexor foot muscles. At 8 days and again at 4 weeks post injection, the severity of leg cramps was graded clinically on the Cramp Severity Scale (0 = no cramps to 4 = continuous cramping severely interfering with daily activities and nocturnal sleep). Eight days after injections, all patients reported considerable relief of muscle cramps with significantly lower Cramp Severity scores. There were no reports of fatigability or weakness of the lower limb and no spread of symptoms to noninjected muscles of the upper leg.

Onset of relief was 4–6 days, duration was 94.2 ± 7.4 days, and follow-up after 5 months showed that cramps had returned in all patients. The authors concluded that BTX-A was an effective, safe, and long-lasting treatment of muscle cramps and fasciculations (Bertolasi et al, 1997).

STRABISMUS AND NYSTAGMUS

Strabismus (disorder of conjugate eye movement) is an ophthalmologic disorder in which there is a lack of parallel movement of the visual axis of the eyes. Strabismus is one of the original indications for BTX-A (Botox).

In an open-label trial of 677 patients with strabismus who were treated with one or more injections, 55% of these patients improved to an alignment of 10 prism diopters or less when evaluated 6 months or more following injection (Scott et al, 1989).

Long-term ocular alignment can be difficult with consecutive and secondary exotropia. Accordingly, 60 patients with surgically over-corrected exotropia were divided into two groups (fusion potential and no expected fusion potential) prior to injection. Of the 30 patients with fusion potential treated with BTX-A, 15 achieved and maintained good ocular alignment and resolution of diplopia. In the 24 patients with no expected fusion potential also injected with BTX-A, 4 patients (17%) achieved and maintained good alignment. Although the remaining patients were not cured, 10 chose to have repeated botulinum toxin injections to maintain their ocular alignment. The authors concluded that BTX-A has a role in overcorrected exotropia and proved especially useful as a treatment given only once for 42% of patients who could regain high-quality stereopsis (Dawson et al, 1999).

In a retrospective fashion, 237 children were treated with BTX-A for strabismus; 163 were included in the analysis. Fifty-four patients were treated to improve binocular vision, with 54% reporting improvement. Eighty-two patients were treated as a postoperative diplopia test or for cosmetic reasons. Eighty-eight percent showed informative post-operative diplopia tests and 44% had more than one injection to maintain improved cosmetic alignment. Twenty-seven patients were treated for paralytic and restrictive strabismus with various diagnostic outcomes (Rayner et al, 1999).

Nystagmus involves the uncontrolled oscillation or jerky movement of the eyeball. The treatment of nystagmus with BTX-A (Botox) has been reported. In four patients treated for congenital nystagmus, a total of 22 injections in six eyes occurred over a 50-month period. All patients were treated at 3–4-month intervals. There were significant improvements in visual acuity in three of four patients with the response consistent enough for the three patients to obtain driver's licenses (Carruthers et al, 1995).

In 12 patients with acquired nystagmus causing oscillopsia and reduced vision, BTX-A was injected directly into the horizontal recti or retrobulbar area. Eight of ten patients demonstrated a measurable improvement in visual acuity with transient ptosis being the most common side effect (Ruben et al, 1994).

SMOOTH MUSCLE HYPERACTIVE DISORDERS

Detrusor-Sphincter Dyssynergia

Detrusor-sphincter dyssynergia (DSD) is an involuntary contraction of the external urethral sphincter during detrusor contraction of the bladder that causes voiding dysfunction and can result in hydroureteronephrosis and renal failure. Patients with spinal cord injuries or spinal cord disease are particularly susceptible to this condition and quality of life and survival are often affected by DSD.

Twenty-four patients with spinal cord lesions received BTX-A in three different protocols. Protocol 1 consisted of four transurethral injections of 25 U of BTX-A (Botox) repeated at 1–3-month intervals; in Protocol 2, four transurethral injections of 25 U of BTX-A (Botox) were given monthly for 3 months and repeated after 6 or 12 months; Protocol 3 consisted of a single transperineal injection of 250 U of BTX-A (Dysport) per month for 3 months. There were 50 transurethral and 35 transperineal injections during 38 treatment sessions. No effects were observed in three patients, whereas 21 patients had significant improvement in maximum urethral pressure during DSD, in duration of DSD, and in basic urethral sphincter pressure. The major difference between protocols was that one injection of BTX-A lasted 2–3 months, whereas the effect of three repeated injections lasted 9–13 months. Transurethral injections also appeared to be more effective than transperineal injections on maximum urethral pressure (Schurch et al, 1996).

In 17 patients with DSD from spinal cord disease, endoscopic injection of 150 U of BTX-A (Dysport) resulted in significant improvement in post-voiding residual volume, bladder pressure on voiding, and urethral pressure 1 month after injection. In five tetraplegic patients, one transperineal injection of 100 U BTX-A (Botox) was administered. A total of 15 injections were given, resulting in improved bladder function in all patients with an increase in functional detrusor capacity and a decrease in maximal detrusor pressure during voiding. Good clinical results persisted for an average of 3 months, although one patient withdrew due to urine leakage (Gallien et al, 1998). These and other findings suggest that BTX-A could become an alternative treatment for DSD in certain patients who are refractory to sphincterotomy or in tetraplegics who are incapable of intermittent self-catheterization (Petit et al, 1998).

Achalasia Cardia

A failure of the cardiac sphincter to relax can result in dysphagia, vomiting, and chest pain. One hundred eighteen patients with esophageal achalasia were randomized to receive a single injection of 50 U, 100 U, or 200 U of BTX-A (Botox). The 100-U group responders received another 100 U at 30 days. Clinical and memometric assessments were performed at baseline, 30 days post-injection, and at termination of follow-up (mean = 12 months). At 30 days, 82% of patients were considered responders without a dose-related effect. However, only 19% of patients who received two injections of 100 U had relapse of symptoms compared with 47% and 43% in the 50-U and 200-U groups, respectively. The 100-U group appeared more likely to remain in remission, with 68% still in remission at 24 months. In conclusion, two injections of 100 U of BTX-A (Botox) appeared to be the most effective therapeutic schedule in vigorous achalasia (Annese et al, 1999).

In a prospective cohort study, 30 patients with classic achalasia received intersphincteric BTX-A (Botox) injections of a total dose of 80 U (20 U in each quadrant). Symptomatic improvement was seen for greater than 3 months in 77% of patients. Of the initial responders, 30% experienced a sustained symptomatic response after a single injection (mean follow-up, 21 months). The mean initial response was 11 months (Kolbasnik et al, 1999). These data suggest there is no difference in efficacy of the two BTX-A commercial products in the treatment of achalasia, and that balloon dilation lasts longer but has more risks involved with the procedure (Annese et al, 2000; Muehldorfer et al, 1999).

Hirschsprung Disease and Chronic Anal Fissures

Hirschsprung's disease is easily correctable by definitive pull-through surgery. However, approximately 10% of patients are continually symptomatic. Internal anal sphincter hypertonicity with nonrelaxation can cause persistent constipation and obstruction in these patients, with anal myectomy being the only treatment.

Intrasphincteric botulinum toxin injections have been evaluated in this population. Eighteen were injected with BTX-A (Botox) 15–60 U into four quadrants of the sphincter. Four patients reported no improvement, two reported improvement for less than 1 month, seven reported benefits for 1 to 6 months, and five reported improvement for more than 6 months. Of the six patients who had no or less than 1-month improvement, three were found to have intestinal neuronal dysplasia. Eight of the nine patients with improvement had documented decrease in internal anal sphincter pressures. Investigators concluded that intrasphincteric botulinum toxin injections are a safe and less invasive alternative to anal myectomy for symptomatic internal sphincter hypertonicity (Minkes, 2000).

The classic treatment of chronic anal fissure is surgical sphincterotomy to eliminate spasm and reduce the pain, spasm, and inflammation that occur with this disorder. However, botulinum toxin therapy has been increasingly popular as well in the treatment of anal fissure, with less likelihood to cause incontinence. In a study of 76 patients with anal fissure, 40 U of BTX-A (Botox) was injected on each side of the fissure. Response was evaluated 7, 30, and 90 days later. All patients not demonstrating a clear improvement at 30 days were reinjected. Ninety days after treatment, 67% of patients reported complete recovery, 25% substantial improvement, and 6% no benefit. Transient gas incontinence (2.6%) and hemorrhoidal thrombosis (one patient) were the only adverse effects. These data suggest that BTX-A therapy appears suitable for initial treatment for anal fissure with minimal side effects (Fernandez et al, 1999).

Fifty patients with idiopathic anal fissure were treated with 20 U of BTX-A (Botox) injected into the internal anal sphincter on each side either posterior or anterior the midline. Two months later, a healing scar was observed in 15 of 25 of the posterior injection group compared with 22 of 25 of the anteriorly injected group. Resting anal pressure was significantly lower 1 and 2 months after treatment in both groups. Investigators concluded that anterior injections improved resting anal pressure and produced earlier healing in anal fissure (Maria et al, 2000).

In a similar study, 69 patients with chronic anal fissure were included in a nonrandomized, prospective trial of intrasphincteric injection of botulinum toxin. Twenty-three received 5 U of BTX-A (Botox) into each side of the anal sphincter; 27 received a total dose 15 U of BTX-A (Botox); 19 patients received a total of 21 U in three injections around the anal sphincter. Patients in the three groups reported pain relief at 1 month of 48%, 72%, and 100%, respectively. Reduction of mean resting pressures was significant in groups 2 and 3. The need for surgery was significantly lower in the last group. These data suggest that intrasphincteric injection of botulinum toxin is a reliable new option in the treatment of uncomplicated chronic anal fissure (Minguez et al, 1999).

Sphincter of Oddi Dysfunctions

Sphincter of Oddi dysfunction (Banerjee et al, 1999) is a common complication of cholecystectomy. An increase in basal pressures of the sphincter of Oddi establishes the diagnosis and endoscopic sphincterotomy is usually indicated at that time.

Twenty-one patients with type III sphincter of Oddi dysfunction after cholecystectomy were enrolled to receive single-shot injections of 100 U of BTX-A (Botox) into the papilla of Vater. Symptomatic responses were evaluated at 6 weeks. Sphincterotomy was performed if patients had no response or recurrence after initial response with botulinum toxin injections. Six weeks following treatment, 55% of patients were symptom free. However, half of the patients who did not respond to botulinum toxin therapy had normal basal sphincter of Oddi pressures and none of these patients was symptom free after sphincterotomy. Investigators concluded that endoscopic injection of BTX-A into the papilla of Vater provide short-term symptomatic relief of sphincter of Oddi dysfunction and can predict whether patients will gain long-term benefit from sphincterotomy (Wehrmann et al, 1998).

COSMETIC USE

Hyperkinetic Facial Lines

Botulinum toxin therapy has been successfully used in the treatment of hyperkinetic movement disorders, painful syndromes, and smooth muscle diseases. The most well-known use is its capability of reducing hyperkinetic facial lines of the forehead, glabella, crow's feet, nasolabial area, platysma, and mentalis regions.

In 162 patients who underwent 210 hyperfunctional site injections with BTX-A (Botox), 95% reported cosmetic improvement of unsightly facial lines or contractions. The best results occurred in the management of forehead lines, followed by glabella, crow's feet, and nasolabial area. Doses for the various regions were forehead, 5–25 U; glabellar lines, 5–20 U; crow's feet, 5–15 U; nasolabial, 2.5–5 U; and platysma, 10–20 U. The effects were seen in 24–72 hours and lasted an average of 3–6 months (Blitzer et al, 1997). In a double-blind, placebo-controlled fashion, 30 subjects were treated with 10 U of BTX-A (Botox) or saline in the glabellar frown lines. The subjects treated with botulinum toxin noted reduction in depth and length of glabellar frown lines compared with control subjects at 4 and 12 weeks post treatment. These data suggest that BTX-A is safe and effective for reduction of glabellar frown lines (Lowe et al, 1996).

SWEATING AND SALIVARY DISORDERS

Axillary and Palmar Hyperhidrosis

Physiological sweating helps maintain core temperature and skin hydration. Properly hydrated palmar skin allows for normal grip and permits tasks such as turning pages of a book or operating machinery. Hyperhidrosis is the unphysiological excessive sweating of the hands, axilla, and plantar surfaces of the body. Approximately 1% of the population is affected by this disorder.

Twenty-eight patients with palmar or axillary hyperhidrosis were treated intracutaneously with BTX-A (Botox) injections at a dose of 2 U/4 cm^2. Sweating abated in 8 of 13 axillary patients and in 5 of 19 palmar hyperhidrosis patients. Sweating was markedly reduced in another 5 of 13 and 10 of 19 of those patients. Two thirds of palmar patients noted a slight and transient reduction in finger grip.

In 243 patients with various forms of hyperhidrosis, BTX-A was injected with an average dose of 30–50 U of Botox or 90–150 U of Dysport for axillae. Palmar hyperhidrosis dosing was on average about 40% higher than axillae injections. One hundred and ninety five axillae, 40 palmar, and 3 plantar patients were treated, with a 100% observed sweating decrease and a duration of effect ranging from 5 to 14 months. A slight decrease in hand muscle strength was noted in some cases that resolved after 2 weeks (Goldman, 2000).

In a randomized double-blind within-group comparison of 11 patients, 120 U of BTX-A (Dysport) was injected subcutaneously into six different sites on one palm; the other palm was injected with saline. Three weeks, 8 weeks, and 13 weeks post treatment, the mean reduction of sweat production in the treated palms was significant. Subjective assessment of sweat production was also significantly reduced at 3, 8, and 13 weeks post treatment. Duration in sweat reduction was 2–5 weeks and three patients reported reversible minor weakness of handgrip (Schnider et al, 1997). These data suggest that Botulinum toxin therapy is safe and effective for palmar and axillary hyperhidrosis (Naver et al, 2000).

Frey Syndrome

Gustatory sweating, or Frey syndrome (auriculotemporal syndrome), usually occurs after surgery or trauma to the parotid gland. It is the result of inappropriate parasympathetic cholinergic innervation of cutaneous sympathetic receptors (Arad-Cohen and Blitzer, 2000).

In a cohort study of 33 patients with severe gustatory sweating, intracutaneous injections of 25–175 U (mean, 86 U) of BTX-A (Botox) were delivered following a 2.5 U per square centimeter grid. A minimum follow-up of 16 months was achieved. The gustatory sweating disappeared within 2–5 days and was controlled in 53.2% of cases with a 20–90% reduction in severity of symptoms. Two patients experienced upper lip paralysis with no other complications. Complications were self-limiting, duration was a minimum 3 months, recurrent symptoms were less severe, and retreatment with botulinum toxin therapy was successful (Laccourreye et al, 1999).

In 45 patients with gustatory sweating, 1.0–2.0 U per 2.25 cm^2 of BTX-A (Botox) was injected intracutaneously. The area of sweating decreased from 17.6 ± 8.6 cm^2 to 1.3 ± 1.6 cm^2 with half the patients subjectively rating the sweating as completely abolished and the rest noting marked improvement. No adverse effects were noted and recurrence did not occur over a 6-month follow-up. Investigators concluded that botulinum toxin therapy is safe and effective and that it can be recommended as the treatment of choice in gustatory sweating (Naumann et al, 1997).

Sialorrhea

Sialorrhea, or drooling, can be a socially disabling consequence of Parkinson's disease, amyotrophic lateral sclerosis, cerebral palsy, and many other chronic neurological diseases. The disorder is not one of overproduction but a result of decreased swallowing activity due to the underlying disease state. In nine patients with Parkinson's disease, BTX-A (Botox) was injected first with 7.5 U in two sites on each side. Eight weeks later they were injected with 15 U in two sites on each side. Six patients reported a 75–85% subjective improvement in drooling. Three patients noted dry mouth for a few days and then no reduction in drooling thereafter. There was an objective 35% reduction of salivary production at the study's completion ($p < 0.01$); the salivary reduction values in good responders being, 44.5%; partial responders,

20%; and poor responders, 33%. Overall, the procedure was tolerated well, with one patient complaining of transient pain at the injection site. The authors concluded that therapy with BTX-A promises to be a simple and effective treatment for the common problem of drooling saliva in chronic neurologic disease (Pal et al, 2000).

REFERENCES

Allergan, Inc. Botox® Prescribing Information. Irvine, CA.

Annese V, Bassotti G, Coccia G, et al. A multicentre randomised study of intrasphincteric botulinum toxin in patients with oesophageal achalasia. GISMAD Achalasia Study Group. *Gut* 46(5):597–600, 2000.

Annese V, Bassotti G, Coccia G, et al. Comparison of two different formulations of botulinum toxin A for the treatment of oesophageal achalasia. GISMAD Achalasia Study Group. *Aliment Pharmacol Ther* 13(10):1347–1350, 1999.

Arad-Cohen A, Blitzer A. Botulinum toxin treatment for symptomatic Frey's syndrome. *Otolaryngol Head Neck Surg* 122(2):237–240, 2000.

Armstrong MWJ, et al. Treatment of facial synkinesis and facial asymmetry with botulinum toxin type A following facial nerve palsy. *Clin Otolaryngol* 21(1): 15–20, 1996.

Arthurs B, Flanders M, Codere F, Gauthier S, Dresner AS, Stone L. Treatment of blepharospasm with medication, surgery and type A botulinum toxin. *Can J Ophthalmol* 22:24–28, 1987.

Awaad Y. Tics in Tourette syndrome: New treatment options. *J Child Neurol* 14(5):316–319, 1999.

Awaad Y, et al. Treatment of childhood myoclonus with botulinum toxin type A. *J Child Neurol* 14(12):781–786, 1999.

Bakheit AM, Pittock S, Moore AP, Wurker M, Otto S, Erbguth F, Coxon L. A randomized, double-blind, placebo-controlled study of the efficacy and safety of botulinum toxin type A in upper limb spasticity in patients with stroke. *Eur J Neurol* 8(6):559–565. 2001.

Banerjee B, Miedema B, Saifuddin T, Marshall JB. Intrasphincteric botulinum toxin type A for the diagnosis of sphincter of Oddi dysfunction: A case report. *Surg Laparosc Endosc Percutan Tech* 9(3):194–196, 1999.

Bertolasi L, et al. Botulinum toxin treatment of muscle cramps: A clinical and neurophysiological study. *Ann Neurol* 41(2):181–186, 1997.

Bhakta BB, Cozens JA, Bamford JM, Chamberlain MA. Use of botulinum toxin in stroke patients with severe upper limb spasticity. *J Neurol Neurosurg Psychiatry* 61(1):30–35, 1996.

Bhakta BB, Cozens JA, Chamberlain MA, Bamford JM. Impact of botulinum toxin type A on disability and carer burden due to arm spasticity after stroke: A randomised double blind placebo controlled trial. *J Neurol Neurosurg Psychiatry* 69(2):217–21, 2000.

Blitzer A, Binder WJ, Aviv JE, Keen MS, Brin MF. The management of hyperfunctional facial lines with botulinum toxin. A collaborative study of 210 injection sites in 162 patients. *Arch Otolaryngol Head Neck Surg* 123(4):389–392, 1997.

Borg-Stein J, Pine ZM, Miller JR, Brin MF. Botulinum toxin for the treatment of spasticity in multiple sclerosis. New observations. *Am J Phys Med Rehabil* 72(6):364–368, 1993.

Brans JWM, et al. Long-term effect of botulinum toxin on impairment and functional health in cervical dystonia. *Neurology* 50(5):1461–1463, 1998.

Brashear A, et al. Safety and efficacy of NeuroBloc (botulinum toxin type B) in type A-responsive cervical dystonia. *Neurology* 53(7):1439–1446, 1999.

Brashear A, et al. A multicenter, double-blind, randomized, placebo-controlled, parallel study of the safety and efficacy of Botox® (botulinum toxin type A) purified neruotoxin in the treatment of focal upper limb spasticity post-stroke. *Amer Acad Neurol* 2001 Meeting Abstract.

Brin MF, et al. Safety and efficacy of NeuroBloc (botulinum toxin type B) in type A-resistant cervical dystonia. *Neurology* 53(7):1431–1438, 1999.

Brin MF, et al. A randomized, double-masked, controlled trial of botulinum toxin type A in essential hand tremor. *Neurology* 56(11): 1523–1528, 2001.

Bryce G, Morrison M. Botulinum toxin treatment of essential palatal myoclonus tinnitus. *J Otolaryngol* 27(4):213–216, 1998.

Carruthers J. The treatment of congenital nystagmus with Botox. *J Pediatr Ophthalmol Strabismus* 32(5):306–308, 1995.

Chang L-B, et al. Use of botulinum toxin A in the treatment of hemifacial spasm and blepharospasm. *Chin Med J Taipei* 62(1):1–5, 1999.

Cohen L, Hallett M, Geller B, Hochberg F. Treatment of focal dystonias of the hand with botulinum toxin injections. *J Neurol Neurosurg Psychiatry* 52(3):355–363, 1989.

Cole R, et al. Double-blind trial of botulinum toxin for treatment of focal hand dystonia. *Mov Disord* 10(4):466–71, 1995.

Comella CL, et al. Extensor truncal dystonia: Successful treatment with botulinum toxin injections. *Mov Disord* 13(3):552–555, 1998.

Corry IS, Cosgrove AP, Walsh EG, McClean D, Graham HK. Botulinum toxin A in the hemiplegic upper limb: A double-blind trial. *Dev Med Child Neurol* 39(3):185–193, 1997.

Dawson EL, Marshman WE, Lee JP. Role of botulinum toxin A in surgically overcorrected exotropia. *J AAPOS* Oct;3(5):269–271, 1999.

Elan Pharmaceuticals. Myobloc® Prescribing Information. San Francisco, CA.

Fehlings D, Rang M, Glazier J, Steele C. An evaluation of botulinum-A toxin injections to improve upper extremity function in children with hemiplegic cerebral palsy. *J Pediatr* 137(3):331–337, 2000.

Fernandez Lopez F, Conde Freire R, Rios Rios A, Garcia Iglesias J, Cainzos Fernandez M, Potel Lesquereux J. Botulinum toxin for the treatment of anal fissure. *Dig Surg* 16(6):515–518, 1999.

Freund B, Schwartz M. The use of botulinum toxin for the treatment of temporomandibuar disorder. *Oral Health* Feb:32–37, 1998.

Gallien P, Robineau S, Verin M, Le Bot MP, Nicolas B, Brissot R. Treatment of detrusor sphincter dyssynergia by transperineal injection of botulinum toxin. *Arch Phys Med Rehabil* 79(6):715–717, 1998.

Gibbs SR, Blitzer A. Botulinum toxin for the treatment of spasmodic dysphonia. *Ophthalmol Clin North Am* 33(4):879–894, 2000.

Goldman A. Treatment of axillary and palmar hyperhidrosis with botulinum toxin. *Aesthetic Plast Surg* 24(4):280–282, 2000.

Hertegard S, et al. Botulinum toxin injections for essential voice tremor. *Ann Otol Rhinol Laryngol* 109(2):204–209, 2000.

Hyman N, Barnes M, Bhakta B, et al. Botulinum toxin (Dysport) treatment of hip adductor spasticity in multiple sclerosis: A prospective, randomised, double blind, placebo controlled, dose ranging study. *J Neurol Neurosurg Psychiatry* 68(6):707–712, 2000.

Jabbari B, Latimer E, et al. Botulinum toxin A and cerebral palsy. *Neurology* 50:A366, 1998.

Jankovic J, et al. A randomized, double-blind, placebo-controlled study to evaluate botulinum toxin type A in essential hand tremor. *Mov Disord* 11(3):250–256, 1996.

Jitpimolmard S, et al. Long term results of botulinum toxin type A (Dysport) in the treatment of hemifacial spasm: A report of 175 cases. *J Neurol Neurosurg Psychiatry* 64(6):751–757, 1998.

Karp BI, et al. Long-term botulinum toxin treatment of focal hand dystonia. *Neurology* 44(1):70–76, 1994.

Kedlaya D, Reynolds, LW, Strum SR, Waldman SD. Effective treatment of cervical dystonia with botulinum toxin: Review. *J Back Musc Rehab* 13:3–10,1999.

Kessler KR, et al. Long-term treatment of cervical dystonia with botulinum toxin A: Efficacy, safety, and antibody frequency. *J Neurol* 246(4):265–274, 99.

Kolbasnik J, Waterfall WE, Fachnie B, Chen Y, Tougas G. Long-term efficacy of botulinum toxin in classical achalasia: A prospective study. *Am J Gastroenterol* 94(12):3434–3439, 1999.

Koller WC, et al. Pharmacologic treatment of essential tremor. *Neurology* 54(11; suppl 4):S30–S38, 2000.

Koman L, Mooney J, et al. Botulinum toxin type A neromuscular blockade in the treatment of lower extremity spasticity in cerebral palsy: A randomized, double-blind, placebo-controlled trial. *J Pediatr Orthop* 20(1):108–115, 2000.

Krauss JK, Jankovic J. Severe motor tics causing cervical myelopathy in Tourette's syndrome. *Mov Disord* 11(5):563–565, 1996.

Kwak C, Hannah P, Jankovic J. Botulinum toxin in the treatment of tics. *Arch Neurol* 57(8):1190–1193, 2000.

Laccourreye O, et al. Recurrent gustatory sweating (Frey syndrome) after intracutaneous injection of botulinum toxin type A: Incidence, management, and outcome. *Otolaryngol Head Neck Surg* 125(3):283–286, 1999.

Langeveld TP, et al. Unilateral versus bilateral botulinum toxin injections in adductor spasmodic dysphonia. *Ann Otol Rhinol Laryngol* 107(4):280–284, 1998.

Liu C-Y, et al. Emotional symptoms are secondary to the voice disorder in patients with spasmodic dysphonia. *Gen Hosp Psychiatry* 20(4):255–259, 1998.

Lou JS, et al. Botulinum toxin A is effective in treating trismus associated with postradiation myokymia and muscle spasm. *Mov Disord* 10(5):680–681, 1995.

Lowe NJ, Maxwell A, Harper H. Botulinum A exotoxin for glabellar folds: A double-blind, placebo-controlled study with an electromyographic injection technique. *J Am Acad Dermatol* 35(4):569–572, 1996.

Lu C-S, et al. Double-blind, placebo-controlled study of botulinum toxin injections in the treatment of cervical dystonia. *J Formos Med Assoc* 94(4):189–192, 1995.

Maria G, Brisinda G, Bentivoglio AR, Cassetta E, Gui D, Albanese A. Influence of botulinum toxin site of injections on healing rate in patients with chronic anal fissure. *Am J Surg* 179(1):46–50, 2000.

Minguez M, Melo F, Espi A, et al. Therapeutic effects of different doses of botulinum toxin in chronic anal fissure. *Dis Colon Rectum* 42(8):1016–1021, 1999.

Muehldorfer SM, Schneider TH, Hochberger J, Martus P, Hahn EG, Ell C. Esophageal achalasia: intrasphincteric injection of botulinum toxin A versus balloon dilation. *Endoscopy* 31(7):517–521, 1999.

Naumann M, et al. Treatment of gustatory sweating with botulinum toxin. *Ann Neurol* 42(6):973–975, 1997.

Naver H, et al. Palmar and axillary hyperhidrosis treated with botulinum toxin: One-year clinical follow-up. *Eur J Neurol* 7(1):55–62, 2000.

O'Brien CF, Seeberger LC, Smith DB. Spasticity after stroke. Epidemiology and optimal treatment. *Drugs Aging* 9(5):332–340, 1996.

Pahwa R, et al. Botulinum toxin treatment of essential head tremor. *Neurology* 45(4):822–824, 1995.

Pal PK, et al. Botulinum toxin A as treatment for drooling saliva in PD. *Neurology* 54(1):244–247, 2000.

Pavesi G, et al. Botulinum toxin type A in the treatment of upper limb spasticity among patients with traumatic brain imjury. *J Neurol Neurosurg Psychiatry* 64:419–420, 1998.

Petit H, Wiart L, Gaujard E, et al. Botulinum A toxin treatment for detrusor-sphincter dyssynergia in spinal cord disease. *Spinal Cord* 36(2):91–94, 1998.

Poungvarin N, Viriyavejakul A. Two hundred and fifty patients with hemifacial spasm treated with botulinum toxin injection. *J Med Assoc Thai* 75(4):199–203, 1992.

Price J, et al. Blepharospasm and hemifacial spasm: Randomized trial to determine the most appropriate location for botulinum toxin injections. *Ophthalmology* 104(5):865–868, 1997.

Rayner SA, Hollick EJ, Lee JP. Botulinum toxin in childhood strabismus. *Strabismus* 7(2):103–111, 1999.

Ruben S, Dunlop IS, Elston J. Retrobulbar botulinum toxin for treatment of oscillopsia. *Aust N Z J Ophthalmol* 22(1):65–67, 1994.

Russman BS, Tilton A, Gormley ME, Jr. Cerebral palsy: A rational approach to a treatment protocol, and the role of botulinum toxin in treatment. *Muscle Nerve Suppl* 6:S181–193, 1997.

Schnider P, et al. Double-blind trial of botulinum A toxin for the treatment of focal hyperhidrosis of the palms. *Br J Dermatol* 136(4):548–552, 1997.

Schurch B, Hauri D, Rodic B, Curt A, Meyer M, Rossier AB. Botulinum-A toxin as a treatment of detrusor-sphincter dyssynergia: A prospective study in 24 Spinal Cord injury patients. *J Urol* 155(3):1023–1029, 1996.

Scott AB. Botulinum toxin treatment of strabismus. Amer Acad Ophthalmol, Focal Points 1989: Clinical Modules for *Ophthalmologist,* Vol VII, Module 12.

Sedano MJ, Trejo JM, Macarron JL, Polo JM, Berciano J, Calleja J. Continuous facial myokymia in multiple sclerosis: Treatment with botulinum toxin. *Eur Neurol* 43(3):137–140, 2000.

Simpson DM, Alexander DN, O'Brien CF, et al. Botulinum toxin type A in the treatment of upper extremity spasticity: A randomized, double-blind, placebo-controlled trial. *Neurology* 46(5):1306–1310, 1996.

Smet-Dieleman H, et al. Botulinum A toxin injection in patients with facial nerve palsy. *Acta Otorhinolaryngol Belg* 47(3):359–363, 1993.

Smith SJ, Ellis E, White S, Moore AP. A double-blind placebo-controlled study of botulinum toxin in upper limb spasticity after stroke or head injury. *Clin Rehabil* 14(1):5–13, 2000.

Tan E-K, Jankovic J. Botulinum toxin A in patients with oromandibular dystonia: Long-term follow-up. *Neurology* 53(9):2102–2107, 1999.

Thussu A, et al. Botulinum toxin treatment of hemifacial spasm and blepharospasm: Objective response evaluation. *Neurol India* 47(3):206–209, 1999.

Trimble MR, et al. Vocal tics in Gilles de la Tourette syndrome treated with botulinum toxin injections. *Mov Disord* 13(3):617–619, 1998.

Trosch RM, Pullman SL. Botulinum toxin A injections for the treatment of hand tremors. *Mov Disord* 9(6):601–609, 1994.

Tsui J, Bhatt M, Calne S, Calne D. Botulinum toxin in the treatment of writer's cramp. *Neurology* 43(1):183–185, 1993.

Varney S, et al. Palatal myoclonus: Treatment with *Clostridium botulinum* toxin injection. *Otolaryngol Head Neck Surg* 114(2):317–320, 1996.

Wang AC, Jankovic J. Hemifacial spasm: Clinical findings and treatment. *Muscle Nerve* 21(12):1740–1747, 1998.

Warrick P, et al. Botulinum toxin for essential tremor of the voice with multiple anatomical sites of tremor: A crossover design study of unilateral versus bilateral injection. *Laryngoscope* 110(8):1366–1374, 2000.

Wehrmann T, Seifert H, Seipp M, Lembcke B, Caspary WF. Endoscopic injection of botulinum toxin for biliary sphincter of Oddi dysfunction. *Endoscopy* 30(8):702–707, 1998.

Wissel J, et al. Quantitative assessment of botulinum toxin treatment in 43 patients with head tremor. *Mov Disord* 12(5):722–726, 1997.

Yablon SA, Agana BT, Ivanhoe CB, Boake C. Botulinum toxin in severe upper extremity spasticity among patients with traumatic brain injury: An open-labeled trial. *Neurology* 47(4):939–944, 1996.

Yoshimura D, Aminoff M, Olney R. Botulinum toxin therapy for limb dystonias. *Neurology* 42:627–630, 1992.

CHAPTER TWO

K. Roger Aoki

Martin K. Childers

PHARMACOLOGY IN PAIN RELIEF

THIS CHAPTER REVIEWS THE PHARMACOLOGY OF BOTULINUM TOXIN TYPE A (BTX-A) with an emphasis on mechanisms thought to be important in pain relief. Key clinical and animal studies are discussed relative to understanding how this product works in a variety of painful conditions. In addition, clinically relevant pharmacological issues regarding the paralytic effects of BTX-A on skeletal muscle are discussed.

Botulinum neurotoxin is produced by the anaerobic bacteria, *Clostridium botulinum,* a rod-shaped, gram-positive organism with spores found in soil and water. BTX-A is one of a family of neurotoxins (designated as serotypes A, B, C_1, D, E, F, and G) which have similar properties (Coffield et al, 1994; Melling et al, 1988). High doses of BTX-A cause degrees of flaccid paralysis (rather than rigid, or tetanic, paralysis caused by a related clostridial protein, tetanus toxin) by blocking acetylcholine release, which is required for muscle contraction, at the neuromuscular junction. Therefore, therapeutic benefit may be obtained by exploiting the pharmacologic properties of carefully administered regional application of this purified neurotoxin (Jankovic and Brin, 1991; de Paiva et al, 1999).

Since there are three commercial preparations of botulinum toxin available worldwide—two based on complexes of BTX-A (Botox, Allergen, Inc., and Dysport, Ipsen, Ltd.) and one on a complex of BTX-B (Myobloc, Elan Pharmaceuticals)—it is important to note that they are not interchangeable generic equivalents (FDA, 2000a,b; Sloop et al, 1997). The units of one product cannot be converted to the units of another product because their efficacy and safety profiles differ. It is important that the physician gain experience with each product to best understand the dose, location, duration of effect, and side-effect profile of the product selected.

ANTINOCICEPTIVE OBSERVATIONS

Botulinum toxin therapy has been reported to alleviate pain associated with various conditions with or without concomitant excess muscle contractions. Early observations in cervical dystonia patients treated with BTX-A suggested that the pain relief was disproportionately greater than benefits gained by decreasing excess muscle contractions (Borodic et al, 1991; Brin et al, 1987; Jankovic and Schwartz, 1990; Jankovic et al, 1990; Tsui et al, 1986). In other conditions, pain associated with myoclonus of spinal cord origin has been treated effectively with BTX-A (Polo and Jabbari, 1994). Tension-associated headaches were also reported improved following BTX-A therapy (Porta, 1999; Relja, 1997; Schulte-Mattler et al, 1999; Smuts et al, 1999; Wheeler, 1998; Zwart et al, 1994).

In a double-blind placebo-controlled trial, Barwood and co-workers (2000) reported profound antinociceptive activity of intramuscular BTX-A when administered prior to adductor-release surgery in children with cerebral palsy. The analgesic effect was so dramatic that the trial was terminated early. Children treated with BTX-A had a reduced need for narcotic analgesics, were discharged earlier, and had better outcomes than the placebo group. In a recent pilot study patients with chronic whiplash-associated neck pain were successfully treated with BTX-A (Freund and Schwartz, 2000). Other reports of BTX-A for reduction of primary pain include trigger point injections (Acquandro and Borodic, 1994), myofascial pain (Cheshire et al, 1994; Porta, 1999) migraine headache prophylaxis (Binder et al, 1998; Silberstein et al, 2000) and back pain (Foster et al, 2000).

However, not all studies have reported positive results (Paulson and Gill, 1996). This variable response to BTX-A therapy appears similar to the early experience with the use of BTX-A in the treatment of movement disorders. As clinicians became more experienced in patient selection, injection sites, and dose, success rates subsequently increased. Therefore, treatment of chronic pain with BTX-A continues to mature with a sufficient number of successes that warrant further investigations.

THEORETICAL/POTENTIAL MECHANISMS OF PAIN RELIEF

Botulinum toxin can affect neurons within the central nervous system (Moreno-Lopez et al, 1994, 1997, 1998). For example, botulinum toxin serotypes B and F and tetanus toxin are internalized by cultured rat hippocampal astrocytes and cleave the appropriate substrate (Verderio et al, 1999).

Purkiss and others (2000) found that neuropeptide release was inhibited by botulinum toxin (BTX-A, B, C_1, F) treatment *in vitro* from embryonic rat dorsal root ganglia neurons (Purkiss et al, 2000; Welch et al, 2000) and from isolated rabbit iris sphincter and dilatory muscles (Ishikawa et al, 2000). More importantly, Ishikawa and colleagues (2000) demonstrated that *in vitro* release of acetylcholine and substance P (but not norepinephrine) from rabbit ocular tissue was also inhibited with BTX-A (Ishikawa et al, 2000). Therefore, based on these *in vitro* and limited *in vivo* data, it can be hypothesized that botulinum toxin treatment reduces the local release of nociceptive neuropeptides either from cholinergic neurons or from C- or A-delta fibers *in vivo*. Accordingly, reduced neuropeptide release could prevent local sensitization of nociceptors and thus reduce the perception of pain. A reduction of nociceptive signals from the periphery could subsequently reduce central sensitization associated with chronic pain. This effect on nociceptive neurons could work in concert with the other well-known effects of botulinum toxin on cholinergic motor neurons innervating extrafusal and intrafusal muscle fibers (Fillipi et al, 1993; de Paiva et al, 1993; Lange et al, 1991; Rosales, 1996; Sellin, 1981).

A preclinical investigation on the local antinociceptive efficacy of BTX-A was reported by Cui and co-workers at a recent meeting of the Society for Neuroscience (2000). A rat model of inflammatory pain was used to demonstrate that subcutaneous injection of BTX-A prevented the classic behavioral pain response to a footpad injection of formalin. BTX-A was administered subcutaneously to the plantar surface of the rat 5 days before the formalin challenge in the same area. The classic two-phase pain response in this model was observed in the rat's behavior. BTX-A produced a dose-related (30 U/kg) inhibition of both phases of the pain response. The highest dose caused a significant inhibition of the acute pain response (phase I) as well as the secondary inflammatory pain associated with phase II. However, the 15- and 30-U/kg doses caused a systemic effect, as measured by the reduced weight gain of the rats.

Further studies with lower doses demonstrated local antinociceptive activity without changes in the rat weights, demonstrating a local effect. Other measures of muscle weakness (behavioral and histological) supported these observations. Taken together, these findings support the idea that injection with BTX-A produces localized pain relief in an experimental rat model.

Preclinical (*in vitro* and *in vivo*) evidence coupled with clinical observations strongly suggest that botulinum toxin (especially BTX-A) may have an antinociceptive effect distinct from its well-known effect on the neuromuscular junction and other cholinergic nerves (Johnson, 1999). Further studies are needed to elucidate the mechanism of this important observation.

MEDIAN LETHAL DOSE

Botulinum toxin's median lethal dose (LD_{50}) has been determined across several animal species, but not experimentally determined in humans. There are two uses of LD_{50} information: (1) to define the biological activity (e.g., units) of a neurotoxin preparation in a standardized manner and (2) to perform traditional safety evaluations in determining the amount of material needed to cause a systemic effect after various routes of administration.

A unit of BTX-A is usually defined in terms of its biological potency. One "mouse" unit (MU) of BTX-A equals the intraperitoneal LD_{50} for a 20-gm Swiss-Webster mouse (Coffield et al, 1994; de Paiva et al, 1993; Mellanby, 1984). Yet, BTX-A sensitivity has been found to vary among different species. The LD_{50} in monkeys has been determined to be 39 U/kg for one of the commercial BTX-A preparations. Based on these findings from primate studies, a human LD_{50} is estimated to be approximately 3000 units for a 70-kg adult. Typical doses for larger muscle groups range from about 60 to 400 total units given in a single treatment. However, due to an inadequate understanding of the complete dose-response curve in humans and a concern for the development of neutralizing antibodies, a relative ceiling dose of 360 units given no sooner than 12 weeks apart is recommended (Brin et al, 1999; Eleopra et al, 1997).

SIDE EFFECTS

Since the mechanism of action of BTX-A is so specific, non-neuro-muscular side effects are uncommon and systemic effects rare. A flu-like syndrome has been reported, but is generally short-lived (Jankovic and Brin, 1991). Other side effects have been reported, but are not necessarily a result of BTX-A treatment. They include muscle soreness, headaches, light-headedness, fever, chills, hypertension, weakness, diarrhea, and abdominal pain.

Muscular weakness, the predominant effect of BTX-A injection, also may be considered a negative side effect when weakness occurs in an undesired area, or when weakness is greater than intended. Therefore, patients should be informed of the potential for either too much weakness in the area injected or in nearby muscles. Clinicians should understand the functional consequences of unintended weakness. While over-weakening the muscles that curl the toes may have little, if any, undesirable consequences, spread of toxin into the muscles that control swallowing (which can occur when injecting muscles near the larynx, such as the proximal part of the sternocleidomastoid muscle) may result in difficulty swallowing (Eleopra et al, 1998; Lew et al, 1997; Lorentz et al, 1990). While clinicians should be generally cautious of this potential negative side effect of botulinum toxin, the following areas should also be given particular consideration.

MUSCLE GROUPS TO INJECT WITH CAUTION

- EXTENSORS OF THE KNEE JOINT (QUADRICEPS)
  Since the knee extensors help maintain the center of gravity in front of the knee, weakening these muscles may result in a

shift in center of gravity behind the knee during walking. This may increase energy required for walking or standing, or even worse, produce an inability to walk.

- ANKLE EXTENSORS

  The tibialis anterior muscle is important in clearing the toe during normal walking. Weakening this ankle extensor too much can cause a patient to drag the toes during the swing phase of gait.

- NECK EXTENSORS

  Although the cervical paraspinal muscles may be a common source of painful spasms in a variety of conditions, weakening this muscle group can produce head drooping during activities like driving, reading, or working at a computer terminal.

- ANTERIOR NECK MUSCLES

  Dysphagia may result from the diffusion of toxin into nearby muscles of the pharynx. Special precaution should be used when injecting the sternocleidomastoid muscle, scalenes, or other structures of the anterior neck. Dysphagia, when it occurs, is often transient, occurring within approximately 1 week of injection and lasting about 2 weeks. Most patients can be managed with a soft diet for a few days. Referral to speech pathology for video fluoroscopy may be warranted if there is concern for aspiration.

RELATIVE CONTRAINDICATIONS

- Conditions of generalized muscular weakness such as neuromuscular disorders, systemic illness, progressive myopathies.
- Patient is hesitant or does not fully understand risks/benefits.
- Profound atrophy of the target muscle(s).
- Aminoglycoside antibiotic therapy (BTX-A may potentiate general weakness).

REFERENCES

Acquandro MA, Borodic GE. Treatment of myofascial pain with botulinum A toxin [letter]. *Anesthesiology* 80:705–706, 1994.

Barwood S, Baillieu C, Boyd R, Brereton K, Low J, Nattrass G, Graham HK. Analgesic effects of botulinum toxin A: A randomized, placebo-controlled clinical trial. *Dev Med Child Neurol* 42:116–121, 2000.

Brin MF, Fahn S, Moskowitz C, et al. Localized injections of botulinum toxin for the treatment of focal dystonia and hemifacial spasm. *Mov Disord* 2:237–254, 1987.

Cheshire WP, Abashian SW, Mann JD. Botulinum toxin in the treatment of myofascial pain syndrome. *Pain* 59:65–69, 1994.

Coffield JA, Considine RB, Simpson LL. The site and mechanism of action of botulinum neurotoxin. In: Jankovic J, Hallett M, eds. *Therapy with botulinum toxin.* New York: Marcel Dekker, 3–14, 1994.

Cui ML, Khanijou S, Rubino J, Aoki KR. Botulinum toxin A inhibits the inflammatory pain in the rat formalin model. Poster 246.2. Presented at the Society for Neuroscience Annual Meeting, New Orleans, 2000.

de Paiva A, Ashton A, Foran P, Schiavo G, Montecucco C, Dolly J. Botulinum A like type B and tetanus toxins fulfills criteria for being a zinc-dependent protease. *J Neurochem* 61:2338–2341, 1993.

de Paiva A, Meunier FA, Molgo J, Aoki KR, Dolly JO. Functional repair of motor endplates after botulinum neurotoxin type A poisoning: Biphasic switch of synaptic activity between nerve sprouts and their parent terminals. *Proc Natl Acad Sci* 96:3200–3205, 1999.

Eleopra R, Tugnoli V, Rossetto O, DeGrandis D, Montecucco C. Different time courses of recovery after poisoning with botulinum neurotoxin serotypes A and E in humans. *Neurosci Lett* 256:135–138, 1998.

Eleopra R, Tugnoli V, Rossetto O, Montecucco C, De Grandis D. Botulinum neurotoxin serotype C: A novel effective botulinum toxin therapy in humans. *Neurosci Lett* 224:91–94, 1997.

FDA Center for Biologics Evaluation and Research—Botulinum Toxin Type A (Botox), Allergan, Inc. Product approval information-licensing action [online] 2000a. Available at: http://www.fda.gov/cber/products/botaller122100.htm. Accessed January 11, 2001.

FDA Center for Biologics Evaluation and Research—Botulinum Toxin Type B (Myobloc), Elan Pharmaceuticals. Product approval information-licensing action [online] 2000b. Available at: http://www.fda.gov/dber/products/botelan120800.htm. Accessed January 11, 2001.

Filippi GM, Errico P, Santarelli R, Bagolini B, Manni E. Botulinum A toxin effects on rat jaw muscle spindles. *Acta Otolaryngol (Stockh)* 113:400–404, 1993.

Foster L, Clapp L, Erickson M, Jabarri B. Botulinum toxin A and chronic low back pain: A randomized, double blind study. *Neurology* 54(suppl), 2000.

Freund BJ, Schwartz M. Treatment of whiplash associated neck pain with botulinum toxin type A: Pilot study. *J Rheumatol* 27:481–484, 2000.

Ishikawa H, Mitsui Y, Yoshitomi T, et al. Presynaptic effects of botulinum toxin type A on the neuronally evoked response of albino and pigmented rabbit iris sphincter and dilator muscles. *Jpn J Ophthalmol* 44:106–109, 2000.

Jankovic J, Brin MF. Therapeutic uses of botulinum toxin. [Review]. *N Engl J Med* 324:1186–1194, 1991.

Jankovic J, Schwartz K, Donovan DT. Botulinum toxin treatment of cranial-cervical dystonia, spasmodic dysphonia, other focal dystonias and hemifacial spasm. *J Neurol Neurosurg Psychiatry* 53:633–639, 1990.

Johnson EA. Clostridial toxins as therapeutic agents: Benefits of nature's most toxic proteins. *Ann Rev Microbiol* 53:551–575, 1999.

Lew MF, Adornato BT, Duane DD, et al. Botulinum toxin type B: A double-blind, placebo-controlled, safety and efficacy study in cervical dystonia. *Neurology* 49:701–707, 1997.

Lorentz IT, Subramaniam SS, Yiannikas C. Treatment of idiopathic spasmodic torticollis with botulinum-A toxin: A pilot study of 19 patients. *Med J Austr* 152:528–530, 1990.

Mellanby J. Comparative activities of tetanus and botulinum toxins. [Review]. *Neuroscience* 11:29–34, 1984.

Melling J, Hambleton P, Shone CC. *Clostridium botulinum* toxins: Nature and preparation for clinical use. *Eye* 2:16–23, 1988.

Moreno-Lopez B, de la Cruz RR, Pastor AM, Delgado-Garcia JM. Botulinum neurotoxin alters the discharge characteristics of abducens motoneurons in the alert cat. *J Neurophysiol* 72:2041–2044, 1994.

Moreno-Lopez B, de la Cruz RR, Pastor AM, Delgado-Garcia JM, Alvarez J. Effects of botulinum neurotoxin type A on the expression of gephyrin in cat abducens motoneurons. *J Comp Neurobiol* 400:1–17, 1998.

Moreno-Lopez B, Pastor AM, de la Cruz RR, Delgado-Garcia JM. Dose-dependent, central effects of botulinum neurotoxin type A: A pilot study in the alert behaving cat. *Neurology* 48:456–464, 1997.

Paulson GW, Gill W. Botulinum toxin is unsatisfactory therapy for fibromyalgia. *Mov Disord* 11:459, 1996.

Polo KB, Jabbari B. Botulinum toxin A improves the rigidity of progressive supranuclear palsy. *Ann Neurol* 35:237–239, 1994.

Porta M. Botulinum toxin type A injections for myofascial pain syndromes and tension-type headache. *Eur J Neurol* 6(suppl 4):S103–S110, 1999.

Purkiss J, Welch M, Doward S, Foster K. Capsaicin-stimulated release of substance P from cultured dorsal root ganglion neurons: Involvement of two distinct mechanisms. *Biochem Pharmacol* 59:1403–1406, 2000.

Relja M. Treatment of tension-type headache by local injection of botulinum toxin. *Eur J Neurol* 4(suppl 2):S71–S73, 1997.

Rosales RL, Arimura K, Ikenaga S, Osame M. Extrafusal and intrafusal muscle effects in experimental botulinum toxin A injection. *Muscle Nerve* 19:488–496, 1996.

Schulte-Mattler WJ, Wieser T, Zierz S. Treatment of tension-type headache with botulinum toxin: A pilot study. *Eur J Med Res* 4:183–186, 1999.

Sellin L. The action of botulinum toxin at the neuromuscular junction. [Review]. *Med Biol* 59:11–20, 1981.

Silberstein S, Mathew N, Saper J, et al. Botulinum toxin type A as a migraine preventative treatment. *Headache* 40:445–450, 2000.

Sloop RR, Cole BA, Escutin RO. Human response to botulinum toxin injection: Type A compared with type B. *Neurology* 49:189–194, 1997.

Smuts JA, Baker MK, Smuts HM, et al. Prophylactic treatment of chronic tension-type headache using botulinum toxin type A. *Eur J Neurol* 6(suppl 4):S99–S102, 1999.

Tsui JKC, Eisen A, Stoessl AJ, Calne S, Calne DB. Double-blind study of botulinum toxin in spasmodic torticollis. *Lancet* 2:245–247, 1986.

Van den Berg, Lison DF. Dose standardization of botulinum toxin. In: Fahn S, ed. *Dystonia 3*. Philadelphia: Lippincott Williams & Wilkins; 231–235, 1998.

Verderio C, Coco S, Rossetto O, Montecucco C, Matteoli M. Internalization and proteolytic action of botulinum toxins in CNS neurons and astrocytes. *J Neurochem* 73:372–379, 1999.

Welch MJ, Purkiss JR, Foster KA. Sensitivity of embryonic rat dorsal root ganglia neurons to clostridium botulinum neurotoxins. *Toxicon* 38:245–258, 2000.

Wheeler AH. Botulinum toxin A adjunctive therapy for refractory headaches associated with pericranial muscle tension. *Headache* 38:468–471, 1998.

Zwart JA, Bovim G, Sand, T, Sjaastad O. Tension headache: botulinum toxin paralysis of temporal muscles. *Headache* 34:458–462, 1994.

CHAPTER THREE

Yuemei G. Corliss

K. Roger Aoki

IMMUNOLOGIC CONSIDERATIONS

THE HUMAN BODY IS CONSTANTLY UNDER THE SURVEILLANCE OF THE IMMUNE system. One of the remarkable features of the immune system is its ability to distinguish friend from foe, ignoring the body's own components and attacking foreign invaders. This feature serves us well and protects us from many bacterial and viral infections. This same feature also presents great challenges for many protein (or peptide) based therapies—how to maintain therapeutic function without alerting the immune system and eliciting immune responses.

Botulinum toxin type A (BTX-A) is one of seven botulinum neurotoxin serotypes, designated A through G, produced by various strains of *Clostridium botulinum.* Currently, two different botulinum neurotoxin products, BTX-A (Botox, Allergan, Inc.) and BTX-B (Myobloc, Elan Pharmaceuticals), are commercially available for therapeutic use in the United States. Due to differences in serotypes and formulations, these products are not the same. Per the Food and Drug Administration (FDA), units of biological activity of one botulinum toxin cannot be compared with or converted into units of any other botulinum toxin or any toxin assessed with any other specific assay method (Allergan, Inc., BOTOX® US Package Insert).

To date, type A is the most studied of the seven serotypes, and Botox has been approved for clinical use in the United States since 1989. It has been endorsed by the American Academy of Neurology and the National Institutes of Health as a valuable treatment for cervical dystonia and blepharospasm since 1990 (American Academy of Neurology, 1990; US Dept of Health and Human Services, 1990). BTX-A selectively reduces muscle hyperactivity without the trauma, general anesthesia, or invasiveness associated with surgery. Also, because BTX-A is injected locally, it reduces the risk of systemic side effects such as dizziness, memory loss, and fatigue commonly seen with oral medications (Brans et al, 1996).

Botulinum toxin therapy is a therapy for many chronic conditions such as cervical dystonia (abnormal head position as well as pain) and blepharospasm; therefore, it is imperative to preserve long-term patient responsiveness to therapy. Over time, most patients continue to respond to BTX-A injections, but a few may appear to have a reduced responsiveness or to have stopped responding entirely. A number of factors such as disease status (progression of the disease), muscle selection (changing of the muscles involved), and therapeutic dosage (adjustment of the dose per muscle) should be examined before any conclusion can be drawn. If a patient has become truly resistant to the treatment, certain tests can be used to ascertain whether the patient has developed neutralizing antibodies against the BTX, interfering with the clinical response (see section below on tests used to detect antibodies or biological responsiveness to botulinum neurotoxin).

The rate of neutralizing antibody formation with BTX-A has not been well studied. However, patients who lose their ability to respond due to antibody formation are faced with treatments that may be less effective or associated with more adverse events (Brans, et al 1996; Dauer et al, 1998). In order to prevent this as much as possible, it is important to reduce the risk of antibody formation with botulinum neurotoxin therapy.

FACTORS THAT MAY INFLUENCE
THE RISK OF ANTIBODY FORMATION

Individual genetic characteristics and overall exposure to botulinum neurotoxin complex protein may affect a patient's likelihood of developing neutralizing antibodies. Some individuals have a predisposition toward antibody formation because of certain genetic characteristics. Although it is not currently possible to identify or control the individual genetic characteristics that contribute to antibody formation, physicians can control the overall amount of neurotoxin complex protein to which patients are exposed.

Overall Exposure to Neurotoxin Complex Protein

One of the basic findings in immunology is that higher amounts of a protein antigen are associated with a higher probability of antibody formation (Rosenberg et al, 1997). Well-controlled clinical studies with BTX-A have not been conducted to characterize the critical factors involved in neutralizing antibody formation. However, the results of several retrospective studies suggest that the fundamental immunologic relationship between protein exposure and antibody formation holds true for botulinum toxins (Göschel et al, 1997; Hatheway and Dang, 1994; Jankovic and Schwartz, 1995).

For example, in one retrospective study, investigators examined the relationship between annual BTX-A exposure and neutralizing antibody formation (Hatheway and Dang, 1994). From a group of 195 dystonia patients containing both responders and nonresponders to BTX-A, complete data on the amount of BTX-A received during the previous year were available for 88 patients. Serum samples from these 88 patients were tested for neutralizing antibodies. The investigators found a relationship between the neurotoxin complex exposure that patients had received in the preceding year and the percentage of patients who tested positive for neutralizing antibodies (Figure 3.1).

Protein Load per Effective Dose

Higher amounts of botulinum toxin complex protein per effective dose may also be associated with an increased risk of neutralizing antibody formation (Göschel et al, 1997; Jankovic and Schwartz, 1995). Data suggest that, in general, patients who receive higher doses may be more likely to develop antibodies. For this reason, it is important to treat patients with the lowest effective dose in order to minimize antigenic potential.

In one retrospective study, investigators compared a group of dystonia patients who tested negative for neutralizing antibodies to those who tested positive (Jankovic and Schwartz, 1995). The 22

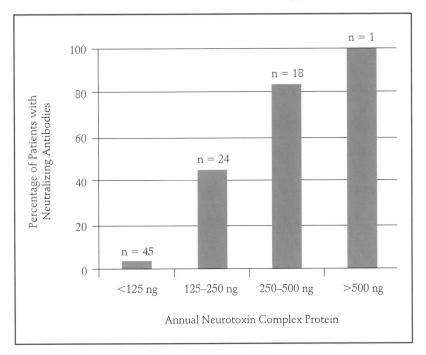

FIGURE 3.1. Relationship between annual BTX-A neurotoxin complex exposure and neutralizing antibody formation (Hatheway and Dang, 1994).

seronegative patients were randomly selected from 1321 patients who were receiving BTX-A treatment at the Baylor College of Medicine; all 22 were continuing to respond to treatment. There were 20 seropositive patients from a sample of 64 patients treated at the same institution who were tested because of inadequate response to injections (n = 60) or at the request of the patients (n = 4). Seropositive patients were comparable to seronegative patients in the average number of visits (7.3, 6.4, respectively), injection intervals (125.5 days, 116.3 days, respectively), and duration of treatment (2.53 years, 2.36 years, respectively).

These authors found that patients with neutralizing antibodies had received higher mean doses per treatment and higher total cumulative doses than patients without neutralizing antibodies (Jankovic and Schwartz, 1995) (Figure 3.2). Of course, when the total dose is increased, so is the exposure to neurotoxin complex protein.

The potential link between neurotoxin complex protein load and antibody formation is also suggested by the ophthalmic literature. Patients

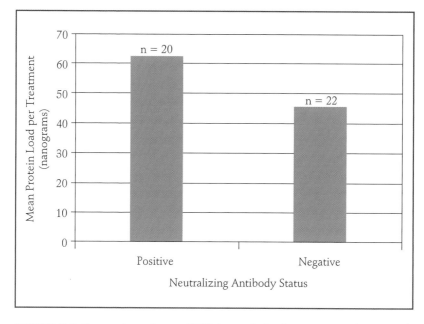

FIGURE 3.2. Comparison of mean BTX-A protein load per treatment* in neutralizing antibody-positive and neutralizing antibody-negative patients (Jankovic and Schwartz, 1995). *Protein load calculated for the original BTX-A product (Allergan) available between 1989 and 1997.

with blepharospasm are generally exposed to less neurotoxin protein than are patients with cervical dystonia because they receive lower doses per treatment session. This suggests that the risk of antibody formation with BTX-A treatment of blepharospasm should be relatively low.

In support of this prediction, one retrospective study of 38 patients treated with BTX-A for blepharospasm or facial spasm found that no patients had neutralizing antibodies (Gonnering, 1988). Although the author does not state how patients were selected for this study, it appears that they were receiving BTX-A injections for these conditions at St. Luke's Hospital in Milwaukee, Wisconsin. In this study, patients had been treated for an average of 99 weeks and had received an average of six treatments. Mean doses per injection ranged from 14 to 31 units, which are much lower than those typically used to treat cervical dystonia (Jankovic and Schwartz, 1995).

In a retrospective observation, investigators estimated the typical dose of BTX-A (Allergan) per treatment as ~150–300 units for cervical dystonia and ~15–80 units for blepharospasm (Borodic et al, 1996).

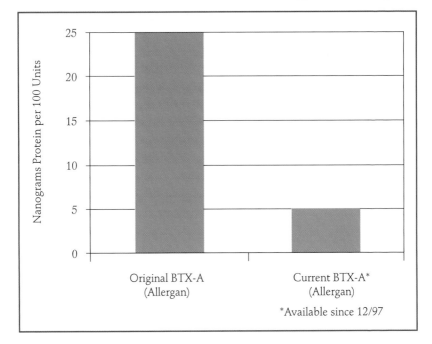

FIGURE 3.3. Comparison of neurotoxin complex protein load of original and current BTX-A (Allergan).

They rated antibody formation as a significant concern in cervical dystonia patients but uncommon in blepharospasm patients. They suggested that the higher risk of antibody formation in cervical dystonia patients was related to the higher doses per treatment and attendant higher protein load. The number of patients, duration of treatment, and method of antibody analysis were not given in the review.

Frequency of Exposure

In the immunology literature, more frequent injections of a protein antigen have been shown to increase the immunological response (Rosenberg et al, 1997). Consistent with this finding, more frequent injections of botulinum neurotoxins may also increase the risk of antibody formation. In one retrospective study, investigators identified a group of 76 patients who had received their first BTX-A injection in 1988; these patients had received a mean dose of 204 units per treatment and had been treated for a mean duration of 23 months. Forty of these patients were available for follow-up, eight of whom had become resistant to treatment (Greene et al, 1994).

In a cohort comparison, the nonresponders had received more frequent injections and a higher percentage of booster injections. Resistant patients also received a higher mean dose every 3 months, which was 311 units compared with 258 units for nonresistant patients. Greene et al. stated in their 1994 publication, "In order to minimize the risk of developing BTX resistance . . . we recommend that physicians wait as long as possible . . . between BTX injections, avoid booster injections, and use the smallest possible doses."

Ascertaining the lowest effective dose for the patients is a time-consuming process. As physicians gain experience with a given product, they may be able to do so more efficiently. The original BTX-A product from Allergan was used clinically from 1989 to 1997. In November 1997, the FDA approved the current preparation of BTX-A, which physicians have been using for the past 3 years. Thus, many physicians have experience in injecting BTX-A (Allergan), which allows them to select the lowest effective dose for their patients and treat at the longest possible injection intervals. This experience may play an important role in delivering the lowest amount of neurotoxin complex protein to patients and in helping reduce the risk of antibody formation.

BTX-A (ALLERGAN) AND BTX-B (ELAN)

The original BTX-A product from Allergan contained approximately 25 ng of neurotoxin complex protein per 100 U. In contrast, the current BTX-A product from Allergan (available since December 1997) contains approximately 5 ng of neurotoxin complex protein per 100 U (Figure 3.3).

As a result of its lower neurotoxin complex load, current BTX-A (Allergan) exposes cervical dystonia patients to approximately 12 ng of protein per treatment based on a mean dose of 236 U (Allergan, Inc., 1998). This protein load is comparable to that of blepharospasm patients who received the original BTX-A product (Allergan). Therefore, it may be hypothesized that cervical dystonia patients treated with the current BTX- A product (Allergan) show a rate of antibody formation comparable to blepharospasm patients treated with the original product.

In a study of 192 cervical dystonia patients with an average disease duration of 11 years who had received multiple treatments with the original BTX-A product (Allergan), 17% had neutralizing antibodies (Allergan, Inc., 1998). The antigenic potential of the current BTX-A product (Allergan) has not been well studied, but investigations are currently underway. However, due to its lower neurotoxin complex protein load, it is hypothesized to have a lower antigenic potential than the original formulation.

As a preliminary test of this hypothesis, a preclinical study was conducted in a small number of rabbits, a species that is commonly used in laboratory immunologic evaluations. Rabbits were given monthly intramusclar injections (3 U/kg) of either the original or current BTX-A preparations (Allergan) (Aoki, 1999). After 8 months of treatment, 8 of 9 rabbits treated with the original product had neutralizing antibodies to BTX-A in contrast to 1 of 9 rabbits treated with the current preparation (Figure 3.4). Although the clinical relevance of these animal data is unknown, they are consistent with the retrospective studies showing a link between protein load and antibody formation. Clinical studies designed to evaluate the rate of antibody formation with current BTX-A (Allergan) are in progress.

The BTX-B product from Elan contained 50 ng of neurotoxin complex per 5000 U. As a result of this, BTX-B (Elan) exposes cervical dystonia patients to ~100 ng of protein per treatment cycle based on the most effective dose of 10,000 units published in three double-blind studies (Brashear et al., 1999; Brin et al., 1999; Lew et al, 1997). According to the BTX-B product insert (Myobloc, US Product Insert, Elan), at 10,000 units, 18% of patients treated for 18 months developed neutralizing antibodies. It is unclear at this time, however, whether the rapid development of neutralizing antibodies in these patients is due to the memory of previous exposure to BTX-A (see cross-reactivity section), the high content of protein in this product, or a combination of both factors.

CROSS-REACTIVITY OF BOTULINUM NEUROTOXIN SEROTYPES

Clostridium botulinum produces at least seven different serotypes of botulinum neurotoxin, referred to alphabetically as types A, B, C_1, D, E, F, and G. Historically, botulinum neurotoxins from different strains of *C. botulinum* were categorized into serotypes based on the distinct immune responses they elicited. In a study published in 1910, Leuchs

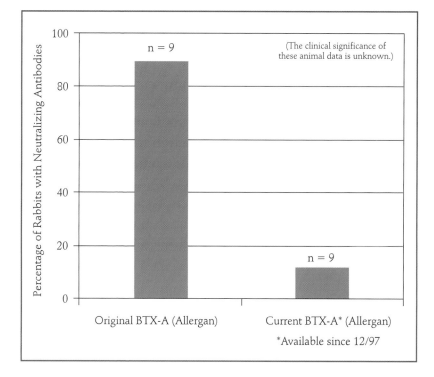

FIGURE 3.4. Antigenic potential of original and current BTX-A (Allergan) in rabbits (Aoki R, 1999). (The clinical significance of these animal data is unknown.)

reported experiments in which he exposed horses to increasing amounts of botulinum neurotoxin gradually to prevent lethal intoxication. When the horses had produced antibodies, Leuchs obtained serum samples from the animals, mixed them with a lethal dose of botulinum toxin, and injected the mixture into guinea pigs. When the serum was mixed with toxin from the botulinum toxin strain that was used to induce the antibodies, the guinea pigs lived. However, when the serum was mixed with toxin from what Leuchs suspected was a different strain, the guinea pigs died. On the basis of this and similar experiments by Burke in 1919, botulinum neurotoxins from the two different strains were labeled serotypes A and B. Later experiments identified other serotypes, such as type F, using toxoid injection instead of active toxin to generate antibodies (Dolman and Murakami, 1961). These studies provided the basis for the classification of botulinum toxin serotypes as antigenically distinct.

These historic investigations were valuable in forming our early understanding of botulinum neurotoxins. Based on these original toxin–antitoxin tests, cross-neutralization was not expected to occur among serotypes following a single exposure of botulinum neurotoxin. However, studies using more modern, sensitive techniques have found both a molecular basis for cross-reactivity and biological cross-reactivity in mice injected with fragments of the botulinum toxin proteins.

Molecular Basis for Cross-reactivity

Investigators compared the amino acid sequences of botulinum neurotoxin serotypes and tetanus toxin, which provide the molecular basis for cross-reactivity (Whelan et al, 1992; Hutson et al, 1994). They found that the percentage of identical amino acids ranged from 31% between the light chains of botulinum toxin types A and tetanus toxin (TeTX) to 56% between the heavy chains of types C and D (Whelan et al, 1992) (Figure 3.5). The higher the percentage of identical amino acids, the higher the chances of having common epitopes.

Still more precise studies have examined the epitope regions (Atassi and Oshima, 1999). Professor Atassi and colleagues identified 13 peptides based on the sequence of the heavy chain of BTX-A that bound to sera from mice immunized with BTX-A. These findings provide evidence that the 13 peptides contained epitope sequences. The investigators aligned the 13 type A peptides with those reported for other botulinum neurotoxin serotypes and tetanus toxin (Whelan et al, 1992). They found that 11 of the type A peptides contained 5 or more continuous residues that were similar or identical to those in other botulinum toxin serotypes or tetanus toxin. Seven of the 13 type A peptides have 5 or more amino acids that are identical to type B. Additionally, tetanus toxin shares 1 identical potential epitope sequence with BTX-A and 4 identical potential epitope sequences with botulinum toxin type B in the heavy chain regions (Atassi, 2000). Thus, there is a molecular basis for cross-reactivity among these proteins. The exact clinical significance of this finding has yet to be determined and clinical studies are currently underway.

Biological Cross-reactivity: Preclinical Data

Two investigators in Maryland conducted a study in which they administered various fragments of the BTX-A protein to mice (n = 5–10 per fragment) using an immunization protocol designed to maximize anti-

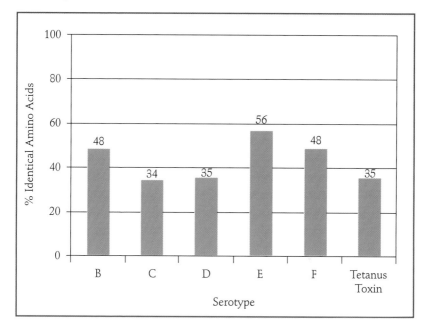

FIGURE 3.5. Percentage of amino acids in the heavy chain* identical to BTX-A (Whelan et al, 1992; Hutson et al, 1994). [*Neutralizing antibodies are thought to bind to the heavy chain (Clayton et al, 1995; Middlebrook, 1995).]

body formation (Dertzbaugh and West, 1996). Serum samples were then tested to determine if they contained antibodies that reacted with any of the other botulinum toxin serotypes. Samples were incubated with the pure type A toxin using an *in vitro* test to measure titer levels. Results showed that virtually all of the 10 protein fragments tested stimulated the production of antibodies that cross-reacted with at least one of the other serotypes.

Biological Protection Assays and Cross-reactivity

The biological protection assays (e.g., mouse protection assay) for assessing cross-reactivity are useful in developing vaccines that must protect humans against a single lethal exposure of toxin (Siegel, 1988). However, these assays do not accurately reflect the therapeutic use of botulinum neurotoxins, which are given repeatedly at lower doses. Due to the different characteristics of primary and secondary immune responses, a single exposure may not be adequate to test for cross-reactivity: the antibody titers to the second noninjected serotype may be too low to protect a mouse against a single lethal dose of toxin. Therefore, the protection assays may not be sensitive enough to detect any cross-reactivity among botulinum neurotoxin serotypes.

In a study using bovine serum albumin as the antigen, Sakata and Atassi (1979) found that cross-reactivity increases when repeated injections are given over time. These investigators injected two rabbits with bovine serum albumin, with booster injections at 7, 14, and 250 days. Samples of antiserum were collected at various time points ranging from 7 to 398 days following the initial injection and tested for cross-reactivity with albumin from other species.

With all of the albumins tested, there was a significant increase in the percentage of cross-reactivity over the course of the study (Figure 3.6). The more frequently the rabbits were exposed to bovine serum albumin, the higher the percentage of cross-reactivity with other albumins.

TESTS USED TO DETECT ANTIBODIES OR BIOLOGICAL RESPONSIVENESS TO BOTULINUM NEUROTOXINS

Various tests have been developed in an attempt to determine whether patients have developed antibodies to botulinum neurotoxins. There is no perfect assay yet available that correlates specific antibody titer with clinical efficacy. However, some of the tests correlate better than others with the patient's clinical response. Clearly, tests that predict the clinical responsiveness are more useful in a clinical setting than tests that do not.

Neutralizing Versus Nonneutralizing Antibodies

All botulinum neurotoxin serotypes are produced as protein complexes that contain a 150-kD neurotoxin protein and one or more nontoxin proteins. The 150-kD protein is the active portion of the molecule. The nontoxin proteins help maintain the neurotoxin's structure and protect it from degradation (Chen et al, 1998).

Antibodies formed against the 150-kD neurotoxin can interfere with, or neutralize, the toxin's activity and are called neutralizing antibodies. Antibodies formed against the nontoxin proteins do not affect biological response and are therefore called nonneutralizing antibod-

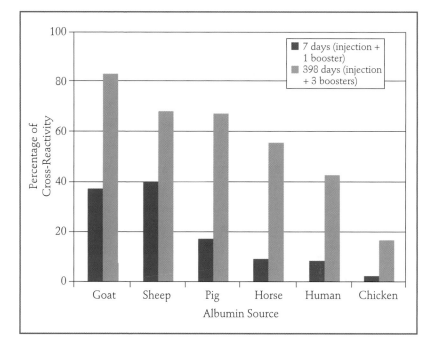

FIGURE 3.6. Serum cross-reactivity in a rabbit (n = 1) immunized with bovine serum albumin (Sakata and Atassi, 1979). The graph shows the percentage of serum cross-reactivity between bovine serum albumin and albumins from six other species.

ies (Göschel et al, 1997). In clinical practice, it is important to use an assay that can distinguish between neutralizing and nonneutralizing antibodies because tests that are specific for neutralizing antibodies correlate the best with clinical response (Göschel et al, 1997).

Frontalis Antibody Test and Unilateral Brow Injection Test

Both the frontalis antibody test (FTAT) and the unilateral brow injection test (UBI) are simple, cost-effective tests that can be performed clinically (Hanna and Jankovic, 1998). They do not test for antibodies directly but instead test the ability of botulinum neurotoxins to interfere with a biological response in the patient—in this case, eyebrow raising (FTAT) or frowning (UBI). Patients are given an injection into either the frontalis muscle in the forehead (FTAT) or the medial aspect of the eyebrow on one side of the face (UBI). If patients are unable to raise their eyebrows or frown in the injected area or on the injected side, it suggests that they are responding to botulinum toxin injections (i.e., the toxin is inhibiting contraction of the relevant muscles). However, if patients are able to raise their eyebrows or frown normally, it suggests that they may no longer be able to respond to botulinum toxin injections (Figure 3.7a,b). In two open-label studies with a total of 74 patients, FTAT results correlated well with MPA results (Hanna and Jankovic, 1998; Hanna et al, 1999). Thus, the FTAT may provide physicians with a simple means of detecting the potential for clinical response.

Mouse Protection Assay

The mouse protection assay (MPA) is an *in vivo* test that distinguishes between neutralizing and nonneutralizing antibodies. In the MPA, patient serum is incubated with botulinum toxin. The mixture is then injected into mice. If neutralizing antibodies are present, they will inactivate the toxin and the mice will live. If neutralizing antibodies are not present, nothing will interfere with the toxin's action and the mice will succumb to the lethal dose utilized.

The MPA is the standard test for detecting the presence of antibodies that interfere with the toxin's action (Hatheway and Dang, 1994). It is the test specified by the FDA, the Centers for Disease Control and Prevention, and the United States military. The results of this test generally correlate well with patient response (BOTOX® US Package Insert, Jankovic and Schwartz, 1995). However, in uncontrolled studies there are individual patients who are perceived as continuing to respond to treatment despite the presence of neutralizing activity. Not all patients who become nonresponsive to BTX-A after an initial period of clinical response have demonstrable levels of neutralizing activity. This may be related to the method of defining clinical response and nonresponse rather than to the result of the MPA assay.

FIGURE 3.7. **A.** Schematic diagram of UBI test. **B.** Effect of BTX-A on a normal responder in an FTAT. *Left:* Normal bilateral eyebrow-raising with the frontalis muscle before BTX-A injection. *Right:* The inability of the patient to raise the eyebrows, despite her attempt, is indicated by the wrinkle-free forehead following BTX-A injection (2 weeks post-treatment).

A

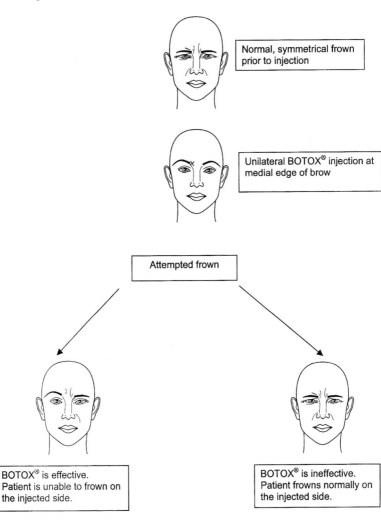

Normal, symmetrical frown prior to injection

Unilateral BOTOX® injection at medial edge of brow

Attempted frown

BOTOX® is effective. Patient is unable to frown on the injected side.

BOTOX® is ineffective. Patient frowns normally on the injected side.

B

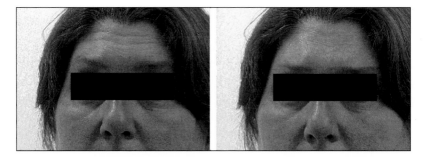

Western Blotting

Western blotting is an *in vitro* test. It combines the resolution of gel electrophoresis with the specificity of immunochemistry detection (Johnstone and Thorpe, 1987). Potentially, it can differentiate the neutralizing antibodies from non-neutralizing ones if the appropriate (reduced) type of polyacrylamide gel electrophoresis is conducted. In this test, botulinum toxin complex is first subjected to analytical separation, so that the positions of different proteins in the gel are a function of their molecular sizes. The array of separated proteins is then transferred from the separating gel to a support membrane. The antigen-containing membrane then will be incubated with a sample of blood serum. Both enzyme-linked and radiolabeled antibodies are commonly used to detect any antibodies in the serum sample that recognizes the antigen. If nonreduced polyacrylamide gel elecrophoresis is conducted, then neutralizing and non-neutralizing antibodies cannot be differentiated.

Enzyme-Linked Immunosorbent Assay

The enzyme-linked immunosorbent assay (ELISA) is an *in vitro* test that can determine whether antibodies are present but cannot distinguish between neutralizing and non-neutralizing antibodies. In this test, a sample of blood serum is incubated with botulinum toxin. An enzyme-linked antibody is then added, which results in a certain color if the serum contains antibodies against botulinum toxin. The results of this test, as conducted with the specified antigen, do not correlate well with clinical response (Göschel et al, 1997). One area for potential improvement of the selectivity of the ELISA is to utilize more specific quantity of neutralizing antibodies in the patient serum.

SUMMARY

Due to the importance of botulinum neurotoxin therapy for the chronic conditions of cervical dystonia, pain associated with dystonia, blepharospasm, and other conditions, it is critical to preserve long-term patient responsiveness. Although the critical factors for developing neutralizing antibodies have not been well characterized, the biomedical and clinical literature supports a link between neurotoxin complex protein exposure and antibody formation. Physicians may help reduce the risk of neutralizing antibody formation and maintain long-term clinical response by treating patients with the lowest possible dose at the longest possible intervals.

When antibodies develop following exposure to one protein molecule, other protein therapies with similar medical effects may be useful as long as their structures and sequences are sufficiently different from the original protein to minimize the likelihood of cross-reactivity. If the two proteins have similar epitopes, then neutralizing antibodies to the original protein may bind to and inactivate the second protein or prime the immune response to react to the second protein faster than in a naive patient. Early tests designed to determine whether two proteins cross-reacted generally used a single exposure to the second antigen. However, a single challenge may be inadequate to assess cross-reactivity, especially with therapies that are administered repeatedly for the treatment of chronic conditions. As the uses for protein therapies expand, it is increasingly important to recognize the potential for neutralizing antibody formation and attempt to minimize it, thereby maximizing the likelihood of patient response over the long term.

REFERENCES

Allergan, Inc. BOTOX® US Package Insert. Irvine, CA.

Allergan, Inc. Data on file—A randomized, multicenter, double-blind, placebo-controlled study of intramuscular BOTOX® (botulinum toxin type A) purified neurotoxin complex for the treatment of cervical dystonia. May 29,1998.

American Academy of Neurology—Therapeutics and Technology Assessment Subcommittee. Assessment: The clinical usefulness of botulinum toxin-A in treating neurologic disorders. *Neurology* 40:1332–1336, 1990.

Aoki R. Preclinical update on BOTOX® (botulinum toxin type A)-purified neurotoxin complex relative to other botulinum neurotoxin preparations. *Eur J Neurol* 6(suppl 4):S3–S10, 1999.

Atassi MZ. Immune recognition of botulinum neurotoxins. Presented at: First Symposium on Cosmetic Botulinum Toxin for the Experts; Vancouver, BC, Canada; Oct. 13–14, 2000.

Atassi MZ, Oshima M. Structure, activity, and immune (T and B cell) recognition of botulinum neurotoxins. *Crit Rev Immunol* 19:219–260, 1999.

Borodic G, Johnson E, Goodnough M, Schantz E. Botulinum toxin therapy, immunologic resistance, and problems with available materials. *Neurology* 46:26–29, 1996.

Brans JW, Lindeboom R, Snoek JW, et al. Botulinum toxin versus trihexyphenidyl in cervical dystonia: a prospective, randomized, double-blind controlled trial. *Neurology* 46:1066–1072, 1996.

Brashear A, Lew MF, Dykstra DD, et al. Safety and efficacy of NeuroBloc (botulinum toxin type B) in type A-responsive cervical dystonia. *Neurology* 53:1439–1446, 1999.

Brin MF, Lew MF, Adler CH, et al. Safety and efficacy of NeuroBloc (botulinum toxin type B) in type A-resistant cervical dystonia. *Neurology* 53:1431–1438, 1999.

Burke GS. Notes on *Bacillus botulinus*. *J Bacteriol* 4:555–565, 1919.

Chen F, Kuziemko GM, Stevens R. Biophysical characterization of the stability of the 150-kilodalton botulinum toxin, the nontoxic component, and the 900-kilodalton botulinum toxin complex species. *Infect Immun* 66:2420–2425, 1998.

Clayton MA, Clayton MJ, Brown DR, Middlebrook JL. Protective vaccination with a recombinant fragment of *Clostridium botulinum* neurotoxin serotype A expressed from a synthetic gene in *Escherichia coli*. *Infect Immunol* 63:2738–27421995.

Dauer WT, Burke RE, Greene P, Fahn S. Current concepts on the clinical features, aetiology and management of idiopathic cervical dystonia. *Brain* 121:547–560,1998.

Dertzbaugh MT, West MW. Mapping of protective and cross reactive domains of the type A neurotoxin of *Clostridium botulinum*. *Vaccine* 14:1538–1544, 1996.

Dolman CE, Murakami L. *Clostridium botulinum* type F with recent observations on other types. *J Infect Dis* 109:107–128, 1961.

Elan Pharmaceuticals. Myobloc™ US Product Insert. San Francisco, CA.

Gonnering RS. Negative antibody response to long-term treatment of facial spasm with botulinum toxin. *Am J Ophthalmol* 105:313–315, 1988.

Göschel H, Wohlfarth K, Frevert J, Dengler R, Bigalke H. Botulinum A toxin therapy: neutralizing and nonneutralizing antibodies: Therapeutic consequences. *Exp Neurol* 147:96–102, 1997.

Greene P, Fahn S, Diamond B. Development of resistance to botulinum toxin type A in patients with torticollis. *Mov Disord* 9:213–217, 1994.

Hanna PA, Jankovic J. Mouse bioassay versus Western blot assay for botulinum toxin antibodies. *Neurology* 50:1624–1629, 1998.

Hanna PA, Jankovic J, Vincent A. Comparison of mouse bioassay and immuno-precipitation assay for botulinum toxin antibodies. *J Neurol Neurosurg Psychiatry* 66:612–616, 1999.

Hatheway CL, Dang C. Immunogenicity of neurotoxins of *Clostridium botulinum*. In: Jankovic J, Hallett M, eds. *Therapy with botulinum toxin*. New York: Marcel Dekker, 25:93–107, 1994.

Hutson RA, Collins MD, East AK, Thompson DE. Nucleotide sequence of the gene coding for non-proteolytic *Clostridium botulinum* type B neurotoxin: comparison with other clostridial neurotoxins. *Curr Microbiol* 28:101–110, 1994.

Jankovic J, Schwartz K. Response and immunoresistance to botulinum toxin injections. *Neurology* 45:1743–1746, 1995.

Johnstone A, Thorpe R. *Immunochemistry in practice (2nd ed)*. Oxford: Blackwell Scientific, 1987.

Leuchs J. Beitraege zur Kenntnis des Toxins und Antitoxins des *Bacillus botulinus*. *Z Hyg Infektionsskr* 65:55–84, 1910.

Lew MF, Adornato BT, Duane DD, et al. Botulinum toxin type B: A double-blind, placebo-controlled, safety and efficacy study in cervical dystonia. *Neurology* 49:701–707, 1997.

Middlebrook JL. Protection strategies against botulinum toxin. *Adv Exp Med Biol* 383:93–98, 1995.

Rosenberg JS, Middlebrook JS, Atassi MZ. Localization of the regions on the C-terminal domain of the heavy chain of botulinum toxin A recognized by T lymphocytes and by antibodies after immunization of mice with pentavalent toxoid. *Immunol Invest* 26:491–504, 1997.

Sakata S, Atassi MZ. Immunochemistry of serum albumin. VI. A dynamic approach to the immunochemical cross-reactions of proteins using serum albumins from various species as models. *Biochim Biophys Acta* 576:322–332, 1979.

Siegel LS. Human immune response to botulinum pentavalent (ABCDE) toxoid determined by a neutralization test and by an enzyme-linked immunosorbent assay. *J Clin Microbiol* 26:2351–2356, 1988.

US Dept of Health and Human Services. Botulinum Toxin. Consensus Statement. NIH Consensus Development Conference; November 12–14, 1990. Bethesda, Md: National Institutes of Health, 1990.

Whelan SM, Elmore MJ, Bodsworth NJ, Brehm JK, Atkinson T, Minton NP. Molecular cloning of the *Clostridium botulinum* structural gene encoding the type B neurotoxin and determination of its entire nucleotide sequence. *Appl Environ Microbiol* 58:2345–2354, 1992.

CHAPTER FOUR

Patrick J. Hogan III

MIGRAINE

THIS CHAPTER EXPLORES THE AUTHOR'S APPROACH TO DIAGNOSIS AND treatment of migraine. Current perspectives on the use of botulinum toxin type A (BTX-A) in migraine are discussed in light of recent preclinical and clinical studies. The author describes an injection paradigm for clinicians considering BTX-A therapy for migraine.

Migraine is a neurobiological disorder that causes intermittent disability in 28 million people in the United States. It is generally thought that about 6% of men and 18% of women currently suffer from migraine that is sufficiently severe to interfere with life activities (Dahlof, 1993; Hu et al, 1999; Lipton et al, 1997; Stewart and Lipton, 1996). Since migraine predominantly affects individuals aged 15–50 years with the peak prevalence occurring at about the age of 35, the incidence of migraine in this age group is even higher. Accordingly, migraine attacks during middle age may have the most severe impact on daily activities.

The magnitude of pain and extent of impairment imposed by migraine are often minimized by those who have not experienced it, or seen as stemming from psychological rather than physiologic origins. These misconceptions can be a major barrier for someone with migraine seeking to receive adequate care. Losing the ability to function because of what others perceive as a simple headache is often distressing to patients, leading to conflict in the workplace and desperation in the medical setting.

Currently less than 50% of those who suffer from migraine symptoms have been properly diagnosed. Of those treated, only about 30% are satisfied with their therapy. It is estimated that migraine costs 13 billion US dollars annually (Hu et al, 1999; Lipton et al, 1997). Such high costs to society could be dramatically decreased by improved diagnosis and appropriate treatment.

DIAGNOSIS OF MIGRAINE

The first step in the diagnosis of migraine is to eliminate the possibility that the patient might have a headache that is caused by another intracranial process such as tumor, infection, or bleeding. A change in the character of a headache pattern or the new onset of headache (especially in the morning) should warn the clinician to look further for other causes. Other potentially ominous symptoms are "thunderclap" onset headache, onset with exertion, headache associated with focal symptoms, and progressively severe headache. Each of these characteristics can also occur with migraine but warrant brain-imaging studies. If the clinician is not certain whether the headache is a primary or secondary headache, pursuing a brain MRI is usually warranted.

Since there appear to be many variations in the manifestations of migraine, the second step in the diagnosis of migraine is to consider atypical presentations that might be caused by migraine (Lipton et al, 1992). The International Headache Society (IHS) criteria for the diagnosis of headaches were generated, in part, to establish standardized patient groups for clinical research studies. In the author's opinion, the IHS criteria for the diagnosis of migraine are excessively narrow for clinical practice. For example, only about 20% of migraine patients have an aura that precedes a unilateral severe headache accompanied by vomiting. Such symptoms are considered to be typical of a migraine presentation. Thus, it would be incorrect to advise a patient that they do not have migraine because they lack classic features such as an aura, unilateral headache, pulsatile headache, vomiting, or light sensitivity.

Migraine characteristically presents as unilateral frontal, temporal, or retro-orbital pulsatile pain. However, migraine may also present as headache in the occipital region or as a bilateral headache described as "steady" or "boring" in nature. Yet clinicians often diagnose patients with occipital headaches or "steady pain" headaches as tension headaches caused by stress and muscle contraction. Migraine may also be misdiagnosed as sinus headache because pain is localized to the frontal and periorbital areas in both conditions. In the author's opinion, episodic frontal or maxillary pain should be considered as migraine etiology unless associated with other features of sinus disease.

The diagnosis of tension headache should be made when there are no associated features of nausea, photophobia, or phonophobia. However, tension headache can cause episodically disabling pain. Experts now recognize that episodic, severe, tension-type headache appears to have an underlying cerebral pathogenesis similar to that of migraine. In recent studies, investigators reported that pain of episodic tension headache responded as well or better to sumatriptan (Imitrex) or rizatriptan (Maxalt) than did pain of typical migraine (Allen and Cady, 2001; Mathew and Mullani, 1998). Some experts now believe that muscle contraction is not the cause of severe tension headache. This idea is, in part, supported by data from BTX-A studies. In these studies, pain relief following BTX-A injection therapy did not correlate with the extent of muscle relaxation (see Treatment below).

In summary, an expanded definition of migraine is *any primary headache disorder that produces impairment in an individual's life.* Treatment can be remarkably similar and equally effective for pain and associated symptoms despite individual variations in symptoms. Headache disorders can still be classified as *migraine with aura, migraine without aura,* and *tension headache,* with the understanding that these conditions are not separate entities requiring different therapeutic approaches.

CAUSE VS. TRIGGERS OF MIGRAINE

A myriad of factors can provoke a migraine attack and vary with each individual. However, these provoking factors are not the *cause* of the migraine event but only a "trigger" of the underlying cerebral etiology of the migraine disorder (Table 4.1).

TABLE 4.1

Migraine triggers

Tyramine, nitrites, or monosodium glutamate
Barometric pressure changes
Change in estrogen levels
Relative hypoglycemia
Bright lights
Cigarette smoke, diesel fume, perfumes
Change in life stress

PATHOGENESIS OF MIGRAINE

The idea that migraine is caused by vasoconstriction followed by vasodilatation has recently been questioned. Instead, some experts now believe that migraine arises from increased sensitivity of cerebral structures in the dorsal raphe area of the brain stem. In fact, this area has been described as the migraine generator. When these sensitized cerebral structures react to various internal or environmental stimuli, a cascade of responses is thought to occur to produce activation of trigeminal nerves. This activation leads to release of pro-inflammatory neuropeptides producing vasodilatation and perivascular inflammation. The consequent activation of nociceptors leads to pain perception (Aurora and Welch, 1998; Cady et al, 2000; Mathew and Mullani, 1998; Weiller et al, 1995) (Figure 4.1).

Once these perivascular first-order neurons are activated, a process is initiated that leads to activation of second-order neurons in the brain stem and third-order neurons of the thalamus. This results in central sensitization that makes the brain hyperexcitable to all sensory activation during migraine including, touch, light, and sound. Central activation also leads to nausea, vomiting, and mood changes. These associated symptoms of migraine can be just as disabling as the excruciating pain of migraine.

In the 20% of individuals who have aura before migraine pain, symptoms are not caused by vasoconstriction as previously thought. It is now believed that once the migraine generator is activated, the

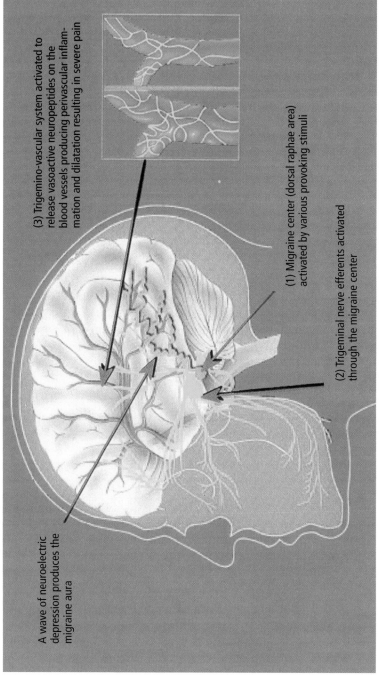

(3) Trigemino-vascular system activated to release vasoactive neuropeptides on the blood vessels producing perivascular inflammation and dilatation resulting in severe pain

A wave of neuroelectric depression produces the migraine aura

(1) Migraine center (dorsal raphae area) activated by various provoking stimuli

(2) Trigeminal nerve efferents activated through the migraine center

FIGURE 4.1. Pathogenesis of migraine.

aura is caused by an electrical wave that spreads across the brain. This has been demonstrated to occur on positron emission tomography (PET) scans during the process of aura (Mathew and Mullani, 1998). If this electrical wave spreads across the occipital cortex, the fortifying visual aura occurs. If it spreads across the sensory cortex, an aura of marching paresthesias occurs.

Although the details in the understanding of the pathogenesis of migraine will be refined by further scientific research, the process described above serves as an excellent working model for discussion with patients and understanding the mechanism of action of medication.

TREATMENT

An effective comprehensive treatment program for migraine includes both avoidance of triggers and excessive analgesics, inclusion of exercise, preventative medication to stop the attack once it has started (migraine abortive medications), and daily medication to prevent migraine activation (migraine prophylactic medications). It is especially important to avoid frequent use of over-the-counter (OTC) and prescription analgesic medication to prevent analgesic "rebound" headaches (Warner, 1999). Most migraine patients still use OTC medications that transform intermittent migraine to chronic daily headaches. Once this analgesic rebound pattern is established, the use of more effective abortive and prophylactic medications will typically be ineffective until the headache cycle is broken.

ACUTE MIGRAINE CESSATION THERAPY

The mainstay for the treatment of acute migraine has become the triptan medications that now include sumatriptan (Imitrex), rizatriptan (Maxalt), zomatriptan (Zomig), naritriptan (Amerge), almotriptan (Axert), and elitriptan (Relpax). Each of these medications is an agonist of specific serotonin receptors along the trigeminal nerve, cranial blood vessels, and brain stem. Triptans stop migraine pain by reducing the release of the inflammatory neuropeptides and also cause some degree of vasoconstriction. Each is effective in aborting the migraine in 70% or more of patients. However, each is effective in a different group of patients. Thus, if one triptan is not effective, it is the author's

---

TABLE 4.2

Examples of preventative migraine medications

ANTIEPILEPTICS: valproate (Depakote), topiramate (Topomax), gabepentin (Neurontin), gabapentin (Gabetril)

BETA-BLOCKERS: propranolol, nadolol, metoprolol

CALCIUM CHANNEL BLOCKERS: verapamil (Veralan, Covera, Calan)

ANTIDEPRESSANTS: amitriptyline (Elavil), nortriptyline, Serzone, Effexor, Remeron

---

recommendation to prescribe another triptan for subsequent migraines. However, some migraine patients do not respond adequately to the triptan medications.

Triptan medications are most effective if used early in the onset of the migraine symptoms (Lipton et al, 2000). Previously, it was common clinical practice to wait until the migraine pattern was established before resorting to triptan medication. Experts now suggest that migraines should be treated before the second- and third-order neurons become activated and consequent central sensitization occurs (Burstein et al, 2000).

MIGRAINE PREVENTATIVE THERAPY

If migraine attacks are occurring frequently or cannot be adequately broken with a triptan medication, migraine prophylactic medication is indicated. The extent that the migraine disorder interferes with the patient's lifestyle is the major factor to consider when deciding on the use of daily migraine prophylactic medication. Prophylactic medications decrease hyperexcitability of migraine generators so that usual migraine triggers will not initiate the migraine process despite exposure to an adequate stimulus. Although some medications decrease migraine frequency (Table 4.2), these are each effective in less than 50% of patients in decreasing the migraine frequency by more than 50%. Success with migraine prophylaxis typically requires multiple trials of various combinations. Despite these efforts, up to 30% of patients continue to have frequent "break-through" headaches with significant disability.

BOTULINUM TOXIN INJECTION THERAPY
FOR MIGRAINE PREVENTION

Plastic surgeons injecting BTX-A to diminish forehead wrinkles serendipitously observed an associated decrease in migraine recurrence (Binder et al, 2000; Lipton et al, 1998). It is unlikely that this decrease is a placebo response, since patients who were being treated for frontal wrinkles were not expecting any change in their migraine pattern. Placebo-controlled and open-label trials of botulinum toxin injection therapy (BIT) using BTX-A for migraine prophylaxis were subsequently carried out (Binder et al, 1998, 2000; Relja et al, 1999; Rollnik et al, 2000; Silberstein et al, 2000; Smuts et al, 1999). These early trials yielded variable results, in part because of a wide range of injection methods and BTX-A doses. However, the author has found the technique used by Binder et al to be successful in his clinical practice.

It should also be noted that BIT has been reported to be helpful for prevention of refractory cluster-type headaches. The author has also observed clinical success with BIT in two patients with otherwise refractory cluster-type headaches (Binder et al, 1998).

WHEN TO CONSIDER BOTULINUM TOXIN
INJECTION THERAPY

Unlike most migraine medications, BIT appears to have the ability to avoid systemic side effects. BIT also has the advantage of potentially producing a sustained effect for 8 to 16 weeks depending on the level of response. In the author's experience, BIT is cost effective in the patient who would otherwise use frequent triptans and daily preventative medications. A formal analysis for a medical insurance system was conducted and demonstrated the cost effectiveness of BIT for migraine prophylaxis (Blumenfeld , 2002).

The author considers BIT for migraine when the disorder cannot be adequately controlled with triptan medication and other preventative therapy. However, it seems reasonable to initiate BIT as one of the first options for migraine preventative therapy. As noted, it is cost effective for the person who would otherwise use daily medication or frequent use of triptans. Many patients would also prefer to have headaches controlled by BIT and avoid daily medication and associated side effects. If BIT is used only for severe migraine disorders intractable to other treatments, the perception of its overall success rate might be diminished, since this group of patients generally has only limited treatment success with any treatment.

MECHANISM OF ACTION

When the efficacy of BTX-A was first recognized for migraine prophylaxis, it was assumed that it was related to muscle relaxation. However, as is reviewed in this book and elsewhere, the efficacy of pain relief from BIT does not necessarily correlate with the level of weakness or muscle relaxation (Freund and Schwartz, 2000; Hobson and Gladish, 1997; Johnstone and Adler, 1998).

A number of the initial BIT studies were carried out for tension headache on the assumption that BIT worked for pain by relaxing muscles and in keeping with the traditional belief that tension headache was caused by muscle contraction. While it appeared that muscle weakness of the cranial muscles after BIT may be helpful to establish that an adequate dose was given, this did not adequately describe the mechanism of pain relief.

It now appears more likely that the mechanism of action can be attributed to dual effects of BTX-A on muscle spindle gamma efferents, resulting in an altered sensory feedback to the migraine generator as well as the ability of BTX-A to block nociceptive ligands at the nerve fiber level (Aoki, 2001; Gilio et al, 2000). It was previously established that other procedures that alter sensory feedback to the migraine generator (such as an occipital nerve block) could break a migraine cycle. Antinociceptive effects of BTX-A have now been experimentally demonstrated in the footpad of a rat (Aoki, 2001; Cui M et al, 2000) and have also been observed clinically in humans (Freund and Schwartz, 2000; Hobson and Gladish DF, 1997; Johnstone and Adler, 1998). BIT will decrease the release of substance P *in vitro* and other ligands mediating pain transmission (Aoki, 2000).

Thus, the author presumes that BIT prevents or moderates migraine attacks by inhibiting the release of peptides in the peripheral trigeminovascular system and producing an adequate feedback onto the migraine generator to suppress the initial activation of the migraine process. This hypothesis is supported by the observation that the migraine aura of cerebral origin is also prevented in those that have a good response to BIT.

There is also evidence that sequential trials of BIT for migraine prophylaxis will progressively be more efficacious. This would be expected as the central sensitization is progressively normalized when control of the migraine disorder is maintained (Burstein et al, 2000; see also Chapter 2 in this volume).

METHOD OF ADMINISTRATION

Initial studies using BIT for headache were done using predetermined techniques and location sites. It has subsequently been observed by many clinicians using BIT that the best results are obtained by directing the injection sites to the areas of most prominent pain. There are physicians who always include the occipital or suboccipital regions in the injection pattern. In fact, the author has observed an improved response in patients (who did not respond initially) by subsequently adding occipital and upper cervical injections to the injection pattern. The success of this technique of including the upper cervical areas is supported by studies with the most promising results. It is suspected that the upper cervical nerve roots are closely interrelated with the trigeminal pathways serving the migraine mechanism.

BTX-A (Botox, Allergan, Inc.) is prepared by the author at a concentration of 5 U/0.1 cc by mixing 2 cc of saline into the 100-U vial of Botox. The solution is drawn up into one or two 1-cc syringes depending on the total dosage administered. (There are others that routinely mix 4 cc of saline for each 100-U vial for a concentration of 2.5 U/0.1 cc. This has the potential advantage of resulting in a greater diffusion distance to reach more trigeminal nerve terminals and muscle spindles.) A 30-gauge needle is used for the injections. There are some clinicians who administer the injections at a superficial depth to allow the development of a bleb at the injection site. However, the standard technique is to administer the solution at a depth adequate to penetrate the muscle area targeted. There may not be any difference in the clinical outcome between these techniques since there is adequate diffusion of the botulinum toxin to affect the structures responsible. Typically, 5 U (0.1 cc) are administered at each injection site, although

2.5 U may be used to increase the area injected and to limit unintended weakness in the supraorbital area. The anterior muscles typically injected are the corrugator, procereus, frontalis, and temporalis. If the migraine occurs only on one side, these muscles may be injected unilaterally (see Figure 4.2b).

The *corrugator muscles* (Figure 4.3) are located just above and deep to the medial eyebrows. These muscles draw the eyebrows inferiorly and medially and produce the vertical wrinkle between the eyebrows. The muscle can be easily injected by gently pinching the medial eyebrow between the thumb and forefinger and directing the needle into this tissue at about a 45-degree angle above the plane of the eyebrows. The injection site (Figure 4.2A) is located 1 cm medial from the midline at a depth of about 1 cm. Depending on whether this is a prominent area of the patient's pain, another corrugator muscle injection can be performed 1 cm laterally to the previous site just above the eyebrow. To avoid brow ptosis, it is important to avoid injections above the medial-lateral aspect of the eyebrow. Injections are typically avoided lateral to the medial third of the eyebrow or about 3–4 cm from the glabellar midline.

The *procerus muscle* (Figure 4.3) is located medially to both eyebrows and can be injected on the right and left aspect of the muscle with 2.5–5.0 U of BTX-A (Figure 4.2a). The needle is inserted at a superficial depth to avoid hitting the periosteum and is directed just laterally to the vertical wrinkle lines in the glabellar region just above the plan of the eyebrows.

The *frontalis muscles* (Figure 4.3) are thin and superficial. To avoid hitting the periosteum, they are injected at a superficial depth by directing the needle nearly tangential to the skin close to the hairline. Two injections are applied to each muscle about 2–4 cm lateral from the midline of the forehead using 2.5–5.0 U per injection site. This is usually done bilaterally, even for unilateral headaches, to avoid the cosmetic problems of asymmetric forehead weakness.

The *temporalis muscles* (Figure 4.2B) can be palpated above the ear lobe by having the patient clench the teeth. The muscle extends more posteriorly than is often realized. This muscle can be injected with 2.5–5.0 U BTX-A about 2 cm above and 4–6 cm posterior to the superolateral orbital rim (Figure 4.2b). Additional injections may be given to the temporal area for a total dose of 25 U or more if the headache pain is most prominent in this area.

Posterior injections are also included for occipital or cervical pain. It is common for migraine patients to have tenderness in the superior

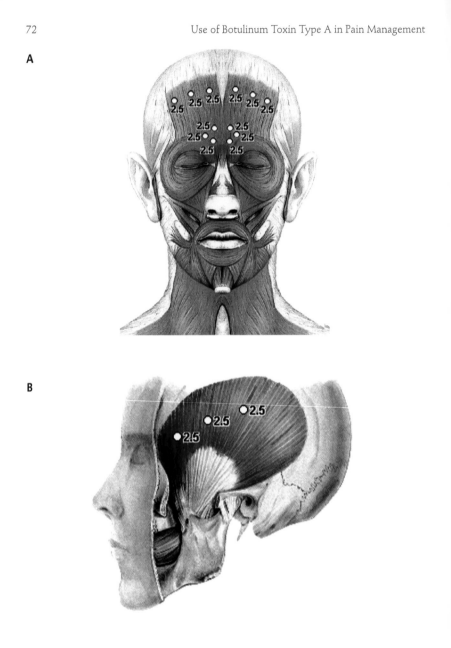

FIGURE 4.2. A. Injection sites for the treatment of migraine in the anterior head using 2.5 U of BTX-A (the author's preferred injection pattern). The pattern and dose of BTX-A used for the individual can be adjusted to the side and location of the most prominent headache pain. **B.** Injection sites for the treatment of migraine in the temporalis muscle using 2.5–5U units of BTX-A. Note that the author uses doses of 25 U or more for prominent headache pain in this area.

C

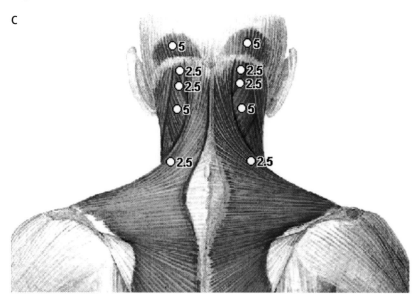

FIGURE 4.2 *(cont.)* C. Injection sites for the treatment of migraine in the posterior neck using 2.5–5.0 U of BTX-A. Note that the author uses doses of 15 U or more in the splenius capitus muscle for prominent pain in this area.

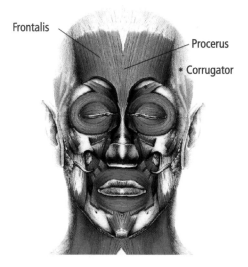

FIGURE 4.3. Deep muscles of the anterior face. The author's preferred injection sites into the labeled muscles are shown in Figure 4.2A. To avoid brow ptosis, avoid injections above the medial-lateral aspect of the eyebrow.

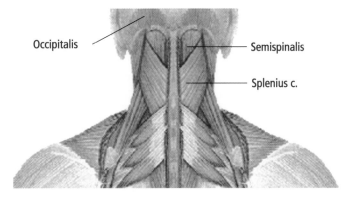

Occipitalis

Semispinalis

Splenius c.

FIGURE 4.4. Deep muscles of the posterior neck. The author's preferred injection sites into the labeled muscles are shown in Figure 4.2C.

angle of the posterior triangle of the neck. Injections are applied in this area lateral to the border of the upper trapezius muscle and medial to the sternocleidomastoid insertion into the *splenius capitus muscle* (Figure 4.4). This site is about 3 cm lateral to the midline of the C3 vertebrae and about 1–2 cm in depth. It is injected with a minimum of 5 U of BTX-A, although doses of 15–25 U are not uncommon depending on the level of pain and associated spasm in this area.

The *occipitalis muscle* is injected 5 cm lateral to the midline and 2 cm below the occipital protuberance with 5–10 U of BTX-A bilaterally. Additional injection sites can be chosen depending on the extent of posterior cervical pain and spasm. Other muscle regions that may be injected (depending on the extent of pain in the posterior and lower cervical area) are the semispinalis capitus and lower trapezius. The *semispinalis capitus* muscle extends along the spinal border and beneath the trapezius and is injected 1–2 cm lateral to the spinal midline in the mid-cervical level. The section of the trapezius muscle in the lower cervical area is superficial and may be injected at the upper edge of the trapezius bulk and again at the lateral base of the neck at a depth of 1 cm.

The author's preferred injection pattern is illustrated in Figure 4.2. Further studies and clinical experience should help clinicians recognize the ideal injection pattern for each patient as well as the characteristics of individual migraine disorders that are the best predictors of a good response to BIT.

REFERENCES

Allen C, Cady R. Effect of Rizatriptan in the spectrum of headache [letter to the editor]. *Headache* 41(6):607–608, 2001.

Aoki KR. Pharmacology and immunology of botulinum toxin serotypes. *J Neurol* 248(suppl 1):1/3–1/10, 2001.

Aurora SK, Welch KMA. Brain excitability in migraine: Evidence from transcranial magnetic stimulation studies. *Curr Opin Neurol* 11:205–209, 1998.

Binder W, Brin M, et al. Botulinum toxin type A for treatment of migraine headaches: An open label study. *Otolaryngol Head Neck Surg* 123(6):669–676, 2000.

Binder W, Brin MF, Blitzer A, Schenrock L, Diamond B. Botulinum toxin type A (BTX-A) for migraine: An open label assessment. *Mov Disord* 13(suppl 2):241, 1998.

Blumenfeld AM. Impact of botulinum toxin type A treatment on medication costs and usage in difficult to treat chronic headache. *Headache Q* 13(1), 2002.

Brin MF et al: Botox for migraine. *Cephalalgia* 20(4):421–422, 2000.

Burstein R, et al. An association between migraine and cutaneous allodynia. *Ann Neurol* 47:614–624, 2000.

Cady R, Sheftell F, Lipton R, et al. Effect of early intervention with sumatriptan on migraine pain. *Clin Therapeutics* 22(9):1039–1048, 2000.

Cui M et al. Botulinum toxin type A reduces inflammatory pain in the rat formalin model. *Cephalalgia* 20(4):414, 2000.

Dahlof C. Assessment of health-related quality of life in migraine. *Cephalalgia* 13:233–237, 1993.

Foster L, Clapp L, Erickson M, Jabarri B. Botulinum toxin A and chronic low back pain (a randomized, double blind study). *Neurology* 56:1290–1298, 2001.

Freund B, Schwartz M. Treatment of whiplash associated with neck pain with botulinum toxin A: Pilot study. *J Rheumatol* 27(2):481–484, 2000;

Freund BJ, Schwarts M. Botulinum toxin therapy for refractory cluster headache. *Cephalalgia* 20:329–330, 2000.

Freund B, Schwartz M. Treatment of whiplash associated with neck pain with botulinum toxin A: A pilot study. *J Rheumatol* 27(2):481–484, 2000.

Gilio F, Curra A, et al. Effects of botulinum toxin type A on intracortical inhibition in patients with dystonia. *Ann Neurology* 48:20–26, 2000.

Hobson DE, Gladish DF. Botulinum toxin injection for cervicogenic headache. *Headache* 37(4):253–255, 1997.

Hu XH, Markson LE, Lipton RB, Stewart WF, Berger ML. Burden of migraine in the United States: Disability and economic costs. *Arch Intern Med* 159:813–818, 1999.

Johnstone SJ, Adler CH. Headache and facial pain responsive to botulinum toxin: An unusual presentation of blepharospasm. *Headache* 38:366–368, 1998.

Klapper JA, et al. Botulinum toxin type A for the prophylaxis of chronic daily headache. *Cephalalgia* 20(4):292–293, 2000.

Klapper JA, Klapper A. Use of botulinum toxin in chronic daily headaches associated with migraine. *Headache Q* 10:141–143, 1999.

Lipton R, Stewart WF, Cady R, et al: Sumatriptan for the range of headaches in migraine sufferers: Results of the spectrum study. *Headache* 40(10), 2000.

Lipton RB, Stewart WF, Celentano DD, et al. Undiagnosed migraine: A comparison of symptom-based and self-reported physician diagnosis. *Arch Intern Med* 152:1273–1278, 1992.

Lipton RB, Stewart WF, Simon D. Medical consultation for migraine: Results from the American Migraine Study. *Headache* 38(2):87–96, 1998.

Lipton RB, Stewart WF, von Korff M. The burden of migraine: Societal costs and therapeutic opportunities. *Neurology* 48:S4–S9, 1997.

Mathew NT, Mullani N. Migraine with persistent visual aura and sustained metabolic activation in the medial occipital cortex measured by PET [abstract]. *Neurology* 50:A350–351, 1998.

Mathew NT, Kailasam J, Gentry P, Chernyshev O. Treatment of nonresponders to oral Sumatriptan with Zolmitriptan and Rizatriptan: A comparative open trial. *Headache* 40:464–465, 2000.

Mauskop A, Basdeo R. Botulinum toxin A is an effective prophylactic therapy for migraines. *Cephalalgia* 20(4):422, 2000.

Petal K. Resolution of chronic tension headache after botulinum toxin treatment of idiopathic blepharospasm. *Mov Disord* 10(3):388, 1995.

Relja M. Treatment of tension-type headache by local injection of botulinum toxin. *Eur J Neurol* 4(Suppl 2):S71–S73, 1997.

Relja MA, Korsic M. Treatment of tension-type headache by injections of botulinum toxin type A: Double-blind placebo-controlled study. *Neurology* 52(6, suppl 2):A203 P03.035, 1999.

Rollnik JD, Tanneberger O, Schubert M, Schneider U, Dengler R. Treatment of tension type headache with botulinum toxin type A: A double-blind, placebo controlled study. *Headache* 40:300–305, 2000.

Silberstein S, Mathew N, Saper J, Jenkins S. Botulinum toxin type A as a migraine preventive treatment. *Headache* 40:445–450, 2000.

Smuts J, Baker MK, et al. Prophylactic treatment of chronic tension type headache using botulinum toxin type A. *Eur J Neurol* 6(suppl 4):S99–102, 1999.

Stewart WF, Lipton RB. Work-related disability: Results from the American migraine study. *Cephalalgia* 16:231–238, 1996.

Warner JS. Rebound headaches: A review. *Headache Q* 10:207–219, 1999.

Weiller C, May A, Limmroth V, et al. Brain stem activation in spontaneous human migraine attacks. *Nat Med* 1:658–660, 1995.

Wheeler AH. Botulinum toxin A, adjunctive therapy for refractory headaches associated with pericranial muscle tension. *Headache* 38(6):468–471, 1998.

Zwart J-A, Bovim G, Sand T, Sjaastad O. Tension headache: Botulinum toxin paralysis of temporal muscles. *Headache* 34:458–462, 1994.

MYOFASCIAL PAIN SYNDROMES

THIS CHAPTER REVIEWS THE USE OF BOTULINUM TOXIN TYPE A (BTX-A) IN painful conditions presumed to arise, in part, from chronic injury and/or overload to skeletal muscle and its associated fascia. The pathophysiology and treatment of myofascial trigger points is described, and a rationale for the use of neuromuscular blocking agents in conditions associated with trigger points is proposed. Clinical data from controlled trials examining the effectiveness of BTX-A use in myofascial trigger points, chronic lower limb pain, and low back pain are discussed.

WHEN TO CONSIDER BOTULINUM TOXIN THERAPY

The use of botulinum toxin in the treatment of a patient with myofascial pain should be considered especially carefully since the approved indications for use of Botox (Allergan, Inc.) in the United States are for strabismus, blepharospasm, hemifacial spasm, cervical dystonia, and related pain. The use of botulinum toxin for myofascial pain is therefore off-label and should be considered only for patients with conditions that remain unsatisfactory or for patients judged inappropriate for more conservative treatment. Before describing specific examples of such treatment, several fundamental properties of skeletal muscle are reviewed and one of the hallmarks of muscle-associated pain, the myofascial trigger point (MTrP) is examined (Mense et al, 2001; Simons et al, 1999).

In general, botulinum toxin therapy for pain management may be specifically appropriate when the pain is determined by the clinician to be dependent upon uncontrolled contractile activity of skeletal muscle. Since all skeletal muscle contraction depends upon the release of acetylcholine (ACh) from nerve terminals at motor end plates, treatments that prevent ACh release will accordingly inhibit contraction of muscle, and presumably benefit the patient troubled by muscle-associated pain. In the authors' experience, when spasticity was sufficiently intense and sustained to cause pain, treatment with BTX-A was beneficial.

Injection of BTX-A should be considered for treatment of pain caused by MTrPs when non-invasive manual treatments were not effective or not available, or when less destructive analgesic medications were ineffective *after mechanical and systemic perpetuating factors have been corrected.* Based on the muscle-weakening effects of BTX-A, injections should theoretically be directed toward the end-plate zone of the muscle. However, when MTrPs are determined to be the etiology of pain, the use of electromyographic (EMG) guidance directing injections at sites exhibiting end-plate potentials (end-plate noise and spikes) is not clear. Presumably, injection of BTX-A should be directed into the end-plate zone, since that is the only part of the muscle where motor nerve terminals are found. However, an antinociceptive mechanism of action of BTX-A (described in Chapter 2) might have important implications in the treatment of myofascial pain. Thus, directing injections toward the area of most intense pain (regardless of the tissue) might be the most effective method. One author (MKC) typically directs BTX-A injections using this paradigm. Future clinical studies are needed to answer this question.

BOTULINUM TOXIN USE IN MTrPs

Some experts believe that myofascial pain syndrome caused by MTrPs (Table 5.1) characteristically results either from an acute episode of muscle overload (Simons et al, 1999) or from chronic and/or repetitive muscle overload. Active MTrPs, which cause a pain complaint, exhib-

---

TABLE 5.1

Characteristic features of a myofascial pain syndrome

- Pain of muscle, soft tissue, and fascia
- Static shortening of muscle fibers and stiffening of associated connective tissue
- Subsequent shortening of muscle and connective tissue, which may lead to further dysfunction including autonomic disorders and chronic pain
- Lack of diagnostic laboratory, imaging, or electromyographic studies

---

it marked localized tenderness and often refer pain to a distant location, disturb motor function, and may produce autonomic changes. MTrPs are identified on physical examination by palpating a localized tender spot in a nodular portion of a taut, rope-like band of muscle fibers. Pressure (usually with the examiner's fingertip) over a trigger point elicits pain at that area and may also elicit pain at a distance from the point under the fingertip. This is known as "referred pain." Another important feature of the trigger point is that the elicited pain mirrors the patient's experience. Applied pressure often garners the response "That's my pain!" Insertion of a needle, snapping palpation, or even a brisk tap with the fingertip directly over the trigger point may elicit a brief muscle contraction detectable by the examiner. This brisk contraction of muscle fibers of the ropy, taut band is termed a "local twitch response" (Fricton et al, 1985; Simons et al, 1999). In muscles that move a relatively small mass, or are large and superficial (like the finger extensors or the gluteus maximus), the response is easily seen and may cause the limb to "jump" when the examiner introduces a needle into the trigger point. Localized abnormal response from the autonomic nervous system may cause piloerection, localized sweating, or even regional temperature changes in the skin because of altered blood flow.

The local twitch response is a transient contraction of taut myofibers that occurs in response to snapping palpation of the MTrP, or in response to rapid insertion of a needle into the MTrP. Animal studies (Hong and Torigoe, 1995; Hong and Torigoe, 1994; Hong and Yu, 1998) and a human study (Hong, 1994) have shown that this response is propagated as a spinal reflex that is not dependent on a supraspinal component. This response is a valuable indicator when injecting an MTrP that the needle has effectively reached at least one necessary target in the MTrP. Demonstration of a local twitch is additional confirmation of the diagnosis. In addition, passive-stretch range of motion of the muscle is limited by pain, and both maximal contraction in the shortened position and maximum voluntary contractions are likely to be inhibited or to be associated with pain.

At present, no routine laboratory test or routine imaging test is available, but the newly developed tissue impedance imaging shows much promise. In addition, two objective tests can be used to confirm the presence of MTrPs. One requires electrodiagnostic technique and the other uses ultrasound imaging. Both animal and human research studies have shown that MTrPs are characterized by electrically active loci that exhibit end-plate noise and often spikes in more active MTrPs (Hong and Simons, 1998). Electromyographers generally recognize these end-plate potentials as normal (Hong and Simons, 1996; Hong and Simons, 1998). However, physiologists have distinguished these potentials from normal miniature end-plate potentials and shown that they represent a pathological increase in spontaneous release of ACh (Ito et al, 1974; Liley, 1956; Simons, 2001). Some data indicate that these abnormal end-plate potentials can always be found in an active MTrP, but these physiology studies suggest that they can also be present for other reasons. Contraction knots (hypercontracted myofibers) to account for the nodule at the MTrP and the taut band were demonstrated histologically in the MTrPs of dogs (Simons and Stolov, 1976).

Injections of MTrPs with botulinum toxin are usually performed on patients with chronic pain symptoms. Some authorities believe that commonly occurring acute, single-muscle MTrP syndromes often revert from active to latent MTrPs without specific treatment if the individual simply avoids the muscle overload situation that activated the MTrPs and proceeds with daily activities within limits that are not painful. This activity tends to actively stretch the involved muscle gently but repeatedly. The recovery of acute MTrP syndromes is expedited and the likelihood of lasting relief greatly improved if the patient learns to perform slow, gentle, active, full range-of-motion exercises specifically for the involved muscles at least once daily. Following injection of chronic MTrPs, the authors consider these exercises essential for optimum results.

The chronic myofascial pain syndromes may have become chronic because the initial, acute MTrP pain was not treated effectively.

Characteristically, chronic MTrPs are chronic because of unresolved perpetuating factors that may be mechanical or systemic (Simons et al, 1999). Simply injecting these chronic MTrPs with botulinum toxin (or anything else) can be expected to provide relief for only a limited time if perpetuating factors are not identified and resolved. Completely eliminating the MTrPs in a muscle with a neurotoxin without eliminating or correcting the muscle overload situation that activated the MTrPs in the first place may only result in that muscle stress activating another MTrP in the same muscle. In any case, since recovery occurs in the injected end plates in a few months (Childers et al, 1998; de Paiva et al, 1999), persistence of the stress that activated the MTrP will likely again activate it. When dealing with chronic or recurrent MTrPs, resolving perpetuating factors is often an essential step to lasting relief.

NATURE OF MTrPs

Research studies indicate that the clinical characteristics of an MTrP can be explained by hypercontracted muscle fibers located at and produced by a region of muscle with multiple dysfunctional motor end plates (neuromuscular junctions). The dysfunction is a markedly excessive continuous release of the normal synaptic transmitter, ACh. The noise-like potentials and spikes that are strongly associated with MTrPs (Hong and Yu, 1998; Hubbard and Berkoff, 1993; Simons et al, 2002) were first interpreted as coming from muscle spindles (Hubbard and Berkoff, 1993). However, EMG studies (Wiederholt, 1970) clearly identified these noise-like and spike potentials as motor end-plate potentials of skeletal muscle fibers. Two recent articles confirm that end-plate noise is significantly associated with MTrPs (Couppe et al, 2001; Simons et al, 2002). Although the EMG literature often refers to these end-plate potentials as representing normal end-plate activity (Kimura, 1989; Wiederholt, 1970), the physiology literature (DeBassio et al, 1971; Heuser and Miledi, 1971) shows that the noise-like potentials result from increased release of ACh, which indicates abnormal function. A physiology experiment (Liley, 1956) showed that end-plate noise can result from mechanical strain of the neuromuscular junction caused by stresses applied to the nerve terminal and clinically from muscle overload. The end-plate spikes, however, are often induced by the presence of the needle and are more likely to appear in more active MTrPs.

Histologically, MTrPs show large, darkly staining, round myofibers found in cross-section in canine (Simons and Stolov, 1976) and in human (Reitinger et al, 1996; Windisch et al, 1999) studies. Portions of myofibers several hundred microns long in the longitudinal sections of canine muscle showed hypercontracted fibers (called contraction knots). The integrated hypothesis for the pathophysiology of MTrPs attributes these contraction knots to the observed depolarization of the postjunctional membrane that continuously releases calcium from the sarcoplasmic reticulum. This hypothesis identifies contraction knots as limiting local circulation because of its sustained, strong contraction of the sarcomeres within the hypercontracted fiber while increasing local energy consumption. The resulting energy crisis should manifest itself in severe local hypoxia, convincingly demonstrated in the German equivalent to MTrPs, nodules of myogelosis (Brückle et al, 1990). The increased tension of involved muscle fibers accounts for the palpable taut band consistently associated with a MTrP. The energy crisis and severe focal hypoxia that was observed to extend for several millimeters could account for the release of substances that sensitize local nociceptors, causing the local and referred pain characteristic of MTrPs (Simon et al, 1999).

An interesting study examined rabbit muscle after a marker (iron deposit) was placed at precisely the location where an active trigger point was identified by twitch response, taut band, and spontaneous electrical activity. Small "c" nerve fibers (most likely nerves that carry pain information) were found in the immediate vicinity (Hong and Simons, 1998). Taken together, these data support the idea that MTrPs are related to abnormal motor end-plate activity and subsequent hypercontraction of the associated myofibers (Cazzato and Walton, 1968).

RATIONALE FOR USE OF
NEUROMUSCULAR BLOCKING AGENTS

If abnormal end-plate activity is responsible for MTrPs, then a powerful rationale exists for the use of neuromuscular blocking agents such as botulinum toxin in the treatment of myofascial pain syndromes and trigger points. The increased tension of muscles caused by MTrPs is clearly not due to involuntary motor unit activity (spasticity) but to the localized contracture of sarcomeres resulting from endogenous end-plate dysfunction. When involuntary muscle contraction (spasticity) is associated with muscle hypoxia, it is characteristically painful

(Mense et al, 2001). Thus it seems likely that any intervention that (at least temporarily) relieves pain by preventing or reducing muscle contractions might predict how a patient would respond to botulinum toxin. Since muscle overload commonly activates MTrPs (Simons et al, 1999) and botulinum toxin is an effective treatment for muscle spasm, spastic muscles with MTrPs are one of the specific indications for botulinum toxin injections. The MTrPs can be a major cause of the pain associated with the spasticity.

However, while trigger point injections or intramuscular compartment blocks by anesthetic agents might predict future response to treatment with botulinum toxin, a problem arises in differentiating the beneficial effects caused by blocking sensory nerves (with anesthetic agents) from the effects produced by a sensory nerve-sparing neurotoxin. While the effect of blocking sensory nerves by injected anesthetic agents lasts no longer than the duration of the anesthetic action, the effect of needling an MTrP (dry or with anesthetic) can also be definitive treatment of the MTrP. Ambiguity arises when a good result occurs because of effective MTrP treatment by needling with anesthetic injection, and also arises when a poor result occurs because there are serious unidentified perpetuating factors that promptly reactivate an effectively treated MTrP.

TRIGGER POINT INJECTIONS WITH BOTULINUM TOXIN IN THE LITERATURE

Studies to evaluate the effectiveness of injections of botulinum toxin into MTrPs are prone to several errors of design that can lead to misleading results. A study that includes placebo injections should use a placebo injection that is not considered to be an effective treatment for MTrPs. If the placebo injection is effective treatment then the study is not placebo-controlled but a comparison of different kinds of treatment without placebo control. There is serious doubt whether injection of MTrPs with normal saline or dry needling are placebo treatments. Injection into an adjacent non-tender site in the muscle should be a more valid placebo control.

Another error that can obscure the effectiveness of any injection treatment of MTrPs is to inject only one or some of the muscles with MTrPs that are contributing to the patient's pain. If only some of the muscles with pain-producing MTrPs are treated, then one could expect that the patient would experience at most only partial pain relief. Poor results could just as well be due to faulty experimental design than to the ineffectiveness of the treatment being tested. Another similar error is the injection of only one of several MTrPs in a muscle so that the untreated MTrP(s) continue to cause pain that obscures the relief obtained by the treatment.

Cheshire et al. (1994) described patient responses to trigger point injections with BTX-A in six individuals with chronic myofascial pain in a randomized, double-blind, placebo-controlled study. Cervical paraspinal or shoulder girdle trigger points in six patients were injected with either saline or 50 U of BTX-A reconstituted in 4-mL saline injected equally in two or three sites. Responses were measured over 8 weeks by verbal pain descriptors, visual analogue scales, pressure algometer, and palpable muscle spasm or firmness. A reduction of more than 30% from baseline was considered a positive response.

Four of six subjects experienced reduction in pain and spasm following BTX-A, but not saline, injections. One subject experienced no change by any variables following either treatment, and another subject responded favorably in all variables after both placebo and BTX-A injections. Onset of responses occurred within the first week following neurotoxin injections, with a mean duration of 5–6 weeks. The authors concluded that beneficial effects of botulinum toxin in myofascial pain occurred through the interruption of muscle contraction, and that a larger study was needed to confirm these preliminary findings before treatment could be unequivocally recommended.

In comparison, Wheeler et al (1998) conducted a randomized, double-blinded, controlled study comparing injections of normal saline with injections of 50 and 100 U of BTX-A at the most tender trigger points in 23 patients with myofascial pain syndrome. The authors found no significant difference in visual analogue pain or disability scores, patients' global assessment of symptoms, or pressure algometer readings throughout 4 months of follow-up. There was a statistical trend toward significant improvement in scores among a small cohort, 39% of the original participants, who were originally treated with BTX-A and then chose to receive a second 100-U injection. The authors speculate that there may be a dose-related effect of the neurotoxin that was not evident in this study, and that further study may therefore be warranted. It is worth mentioning, however, that the group receiving second injections contained significantly fewer patients with work-related injuries than the control group.

IDENTIFYING MYOFASCIAL PAIN SYNDROMES FOR BOTULINUM TOXIN THERAPY

Although any of the approximately 500 muscles in the body can develop myofascial pain caused by MTrPs and therefore could, when indicated, benefit from accurately placed injection with botulinum toxin, only a limited number of sites have been reported in the literature to date. Factors that might identify a pain syndrome of myofascial origin as potentially responding favorably to botulinum toxin injections include muscle hypertrophy, neurogenic and/or vascular compression, anatomic localization that isolates the target muscle from other structures, and more than one outcome measure to determine efficacy of treatment. Under these criteria, piriformis muscle syndrome and thoracic outlet syndrome appear to qualify.

CHRONIC LOWER LIMB PAIN

Chronic lower limb pain (piriformis muscle syndrome) (Hallin, 1983; Simons and Travell, 1983c; Solheim et al, 1981; Travell and Simons, 1992) is a myofascial pain condition that presents with seemingly bizarre symptoms. Patients are typically female, have a recent history of trauma to the buttocks or pelvis (usually from a fall), and describe a deep-seated pain in the buttocks and hip, with radiation into the thigh or even into the leg and foot. These characteristic signs and symptoms are sometimes caused by pain referred from piriformis MTrPs (Parziale et al, 1996; Simons and Travell, 1983a, 1983b, 1983c) and sometimes caused by compression of the sciatic nerve between the bony rim of the foramen and a hypertrophied piriformis muscle (Chen and Wan, 1992; Travell and Simons, 1992) (Figure 5.1). The nodular MTrP and its taut band can provide the increased muscle bulk and tension. Pain in these patients may come from both the nerve entrapment and the referred pain from the piriformis MTrPs. An additional source of pain in these patients is the tendency for compression of motor nerves to activate MTrPs in the muscles supplied by that nerve. Although some clinicians feel that this diagnosis is controversial (especially if they never palpated an MTrP and must take the diagnosis on faith), numerous peer-reviewed articles clearly define clinical, anatomical, and electrophysiological evidence for this distinct condition causing low back and leg pain (Fishman and Zybert, 1992; Hallin 1983; Jankiewicz, 1991; Julsrud,

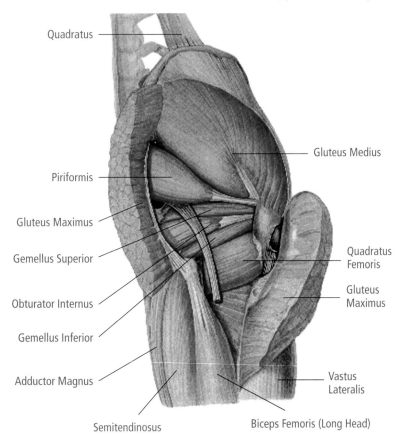

FIGURE 5.1. Muscles of the right hip, deep view.

1989; Noftal, 1988; Simons and Travell, 1983; Solheim et al, 1981; Steiner et al, 1987).

On clinical examination, deep pressure over the buttocks at a point midway between the sacrum and greater trochanter of the hip will reproduce the patient's pain complaint. Full-stretch range of motion of the piriformis muscle is limited by pain. Since the piriformis muscle is so deep, direct palpation of this trigger point can only be properly performed by rectal or vaginal examination and requires unusually long fingers. Deep along the posterior-lateral portion of the rectal (or vaginal) vault, cephalad to the levator ani muscle, palpation of the intrapelvic attachment area of the taut band of the trigger point elicits pain at the site of compression and refers pain either into the thigh and/or down the leg. However, the intrapelvic examination alone can only barely reach the attachment region of the piriformis and may therefore be palpating first sacral nerve root tenderness and secondary piriformis attachment TrP tenderness. The attachment of the muscle at the greater trochanter is prone to be more involved and tender and is readily available for palpation (*note:* muscle fiber attachments converge there, but fan out across the sacrum). It is very useful to identify both the central MTrP tenderness in the region of the mid-belly and also the attachment tenderness at both ends. This strengthens the MTrP diagnosis greatly.

Beatty's maneuver has been described to elicit pain in this condition as well (Beatty, 1994). It requires that the patient lie on the non-painful side, and abducts the thigh by moving the painful leg off the table. This maneuver effectively contracts the piriformis muscle and should reproduce patient's pain in the buttocks. However, contraction of muscles with TrPs appears to be most painful when the muscle is voluntarily contracted in the shortened position. If the enthesopathy is sensitive enough, the muscle hurts when forcefully loaded in any position, but particularly in the shortened position, especially if the muscle is also contracted voluntarily.

Alternatively, to stretch the piriformis muscle one must internally rotate and adduct the thigh at the hip. The most effective way to put this muscle on stretch is to have the patient lie on the nonpainful side, flex the hip to 90 degrees and adduct it by allowing it to drop over the edge of the table. This is also a very effective treatment position for contact–relax manual therapy (Dobrusin, 1989; Simons et al, 1999; Steiner et al, 1987).

However, since the syndrome commonly includes sciatic nerve compression at the level of the hip, other causes of sciatica should be ruled out (such as a herniated lumbar disc). One helpful diagnostic aid is electromyography. In the case of sciatic neuropathy at the level of the nerve root in the back, the EMG exam may reveal abnormal spontaneous electrical activity in the extensor muscles of the back, while in piriformis syndrome no such abnormal electrical activity should be seen in the back muscles (LaBan et al, 1982), since the site of nerve compression is distal to the nerve root. Other investigators (Fishman and Zybert, 1992) have reported that H-wave studies are delayed when comparing the patient's extended painful leg with the same leg in a position of adduction, internal rotation, and flexion. Conduction may be delayed when the muscle is at its thickest in the shortened position, especially if the muscle is also contracted voluntarily.

DIAGNOSIS OF PIRIFORMIS MUSCLE SYNDROME

The syndrome described above may be caused by two distinct etiologies (piriformis MTrP syndrome, and a condition complicated by sciatic nerve entrapment). Accordingly, the clinician should evaluate patients with this putative diagnosis for other causes of sciatic neuropathy from compression at the level of the spine (such as a herniated disc, or space-occupying lesion). Imaging studies, such as CT or MRI, may also be considered to rule out other potential sources of compression at or near the sciatic notch, such as intrapelvic abscess, occult tumor, or hematoma (Chen 1992; Kinahan and Douglas, 1995; Ku et al, 1995). Additionally, all the criteria described above should be met to accurately identify and determine the location of the MTrP. Taken together, these clinical findings, electrodiagnostic data, and imaging studies should enable the clinician to reach an accurate diagnosis.

WHEN TO CONSIDER BOTULINUM TOXIN

In some cases, conservative treatment of piriformis syndrome fails, and local injections of anesthetics and/or steroids may be considered. Surgical resection of the piriformis muscle is an additional option (Kao and Voolson, 1992; Lu et al, 1985; Sayson et al, 1994). However, some patients may gain short-term benefits from local trigger point injections into the muscle but remain refractory to other treatment for long-term pain control. This subset of patients might benefit from botulinum toxin treatment, especially if the piriformis muscle shows electromyographic evidence of involuntary muscle contraction (spasm). When injecting MTrPs in the piriformis muscle, they are hard to localize accurately in such a deep muscle and are located in the end-plate zone in the midbelly region of the muscle. In this case, use of EMG guidance to inject the neurotoxin specifically where end-plate potentials are observed will ensure optimal placement of the product (Childers et al, in press). Since all or part of the sciatic nerve may occasionally traverse this part of the muscle, this use of EMG guidance is of additional importance.

To examine the effectiveness of intramuscular BTX-A injections as a treatment for piriformis muscle syndrome, one of the authors (MKC) conducted a double-blind, single-group, crossover pilot study of nine women with chronic buttock, hip, and lower limb pain with-

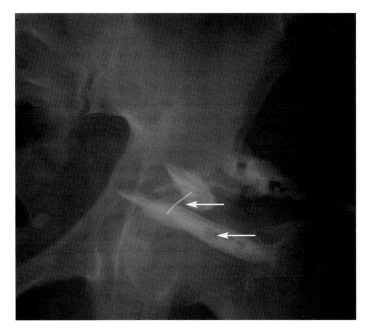

FIGURE 5.2. Anteroposterior radiograph of the right hemipelvis following 3-mL injection of radiotracer dye into the piriformis muscle in a patient with chronic lower limb pain (piriformis syndrome). A 20-gauge, 5 ½-inch needle *(upper arrow)* was directed slightly lateral to medial, and inserted to the depth of the ileum. Contrast dye *(lower arrow)* extends from the greater trochanter of the hip toward the caudal sacrum. Insertion of the needle reproduced the patient's usual pain. The dye pattern (slightly superior) resulted from a previous attempt at needle placement targeted for the piriformis muscle.

out evidence of lumbar disc herniation or nerve root impingement (Childers et al, 2001, under revision). Both fluoroscopic (Figure 5.2) and EMG guidance was used for unilateral intramuscular piriformis injection (Figure 5.3) with 100 U BTX-A and compared with similar injection with vehicle alone. Visual analogue pain scales (VASs) of pain intensity, distress, spasm, and interference with activities were used as outcome measures. Results demonstrated that no differences in mean VASs were detected between groups at baseline or after injection with vehicle. However, decreases (p < 0.05) were observed between baseline and post-BTX-A injection mean VASs, but only in one of four categories (interference with activities). VASs from every time point (days) were also compared with the average baseline VASs.

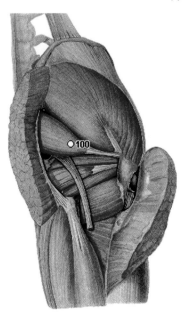

FIGURE 5.3. The author's injection site (100 U BTX-A) for the right piriformis muscle. Note that the needle insertion site is lateral to the widest portion of the muscle to avoid inadvertent needle contact with the sciatic nerve. The needle is angled toward the midline of the body. Presumably, neurotoxin injections spread similarly to the radiotracer dye pattern shown in Figure 5.2.

After injection with vehicle, decreases ($p < 0.05$) were detected, but only in one of the four categories (distress). In comparison, after injection with BTX-A, decreases ($p < 0.05$) were observed in all VAS categories. These data suggest that intramuscular piriformis injections with 100 U BTX-A can reduce nonradicular lower limb pain to a greater extent than similar injections with vehicle alone.

THORACIC OUTLET SYNDROME

Thoracic outlet syndrome (Fricton, 1989; Simons et al, 1999; Sucher, 1990) is a myofascial pain syndrome involving compression of the nerves of the brachial plexus and/or the vessels (subclavian artery and vein) of the upper limb. Compression occurs as the vulnerable structures pass over or adjacent to the first rib as they exit the thoracic cavity or neck region (Fig. 5.4). Since the thoracic outlet is bounded by the anterior and middle scalene muscles, the first rib, the clavicle, and (inferiorly) by the tendon of the pectoralis minor muscle, increased tension of these two scalene muscles elevates the first rib, or hypertrophy (enlargement) of these muscles can cause or contribute to signs and symptoms of this syndrome (Table 5.2; Simons et al, 1999).

SIGNS AND SYMPTOMS

Signs and symptoms of thoracic outlet syndrome include painful sensations in the shoulder and ulnar nerve distribution of the hand. In a clinical maneuver, Adson's test, the patient turns his head to the involved side, and holds a beep breath while raising the chin (Dobrusin, 1989; Pang and Wessel, 1988; Sucher, 1990). The examiner palpates the radial pulse. A positive test is determined in the individual whose pulse diminishes and in whom pain is reproduced during this maneuver.

A similar clinical maneuver, known as "Roos' test" requires the patient to abduct the shoulders 90 degrees, flex the elbows 90 degrees, and open/close his hands slowly for 3 minutes (Pang and Wessel, 1988; Urschel, 1972). The examiner observes the patient for hand pallor, diminished pulses, and ulnar dysesthesias (all positive for thoracic outlet syndrome).

Scalene MTrPs are found by examining the head and neck for painful restriction of side-bending of the head to the opposite side, directly and also slightly posteriorly. Also, one should examine the digitations of the anterior and middle scalene muscles for tender spots in taut bands. Other causes of compression (besides muscle hypertrophy) in the thoracic outlet should be considered since the thoracic outlet is an enclosed, relatively small space. This includes anything that might narrow the space or cause swelling and edema of any of the associated structures, such as

- fractured clavicle,
- cervical rib,
- tumor within the thoracic outlet,
- movements that compress the thoracic outlet (shoulder hyperabduction), and
- paradoxical or chest breathing (vs. coordinated diaphragm breathing), an aggravating factor for scalene MTrPs (Simons et al, 1999).

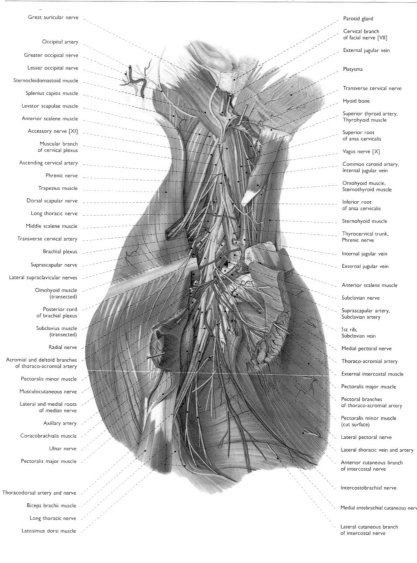

Great auricular nerve
Occipital artery
Greater occipital nerve
Lesser occipital nerve
Sternocleidomastoid muscle
Splenius capitis muscle
Levator scapulae muscle
Anterior scalene muscle
Accessory nerve [XI]
Muscular branch of cervical plexus
Ascending cervical artery
Phrenic nerve
Trapezius muscle
Dorsal scapular nerve
Long thoracic nerve
Middle scalene muscle
Transverse cervical artery
Brachial plexus
Suprascapular nerve
Lateral supraclavicular nerves
Omohyoid muscle (transected)
Posterior cord of brachial plexus
Subclavius muscle (transected)
Radial nerve
Acromial and deltoid branches of thoraco-acromial artery
Pectoralis minor muscle
Musculocutaneous nerve
Lateral and medial roots of median nerve
Axillary artery
Coracobrachialis muscle
Ulnar nerve
Pectoralis major muscle
Thoracodorsal artery and nerve
Biceps brachii muscle
Long thoracic nerve
Latissimus dorsi muscle

Parotid gland
Cervical branch of facial nerve [VII]
External jugular vein
Platysma
Transverse cervical nerve
Hyoid bone
Superior thyroid artery, Thyrohyoid muscle
Superior root of ansa cervicalis
Vagus nerve [X]
Common carotid artery, Internal jugular vein
Omohyoid muscle, Sternothyroid muscle
Inferior root of ansa cervicalis
Sternohyoid muscle
Thyrocervical trunk, Phrenic nerve
Internal jugular vein
External jugular vein
Anterior scalene muscle
Subclavian nerve
Suprascapular artery, Subclavian artery
1st rib, Subclavian vein
Medial pectoral nerve
Thoraco-acromial artery
External intercostal muscle
Pectoralis major muscle
Pectoral branches of thoraco-acromial artery
Pectoralis minor muscle (cut surface)
Lateral pectoral nerve
Lateral thoracic vein and artery
Anterior cutaneous branch of intercostal nerve
Intercostobrachial nerve
Medial antebrachial cutaneous nerve
Lateral cutaneous branch of intercostal nerve

FIGURE 5.4. Relationship of anatomical structures in and around the thoracic outlet. Notice the close proximity of vessels and nerves to the scalene muscles. Because
of the risk of inadvertant contact between an injection needle and vessels or nerves,
the clinician should take great care when attempting to inject the scalene muscles.
Injections in this region should be guided by computed tomography, fluoroscopy,
or electromyography.

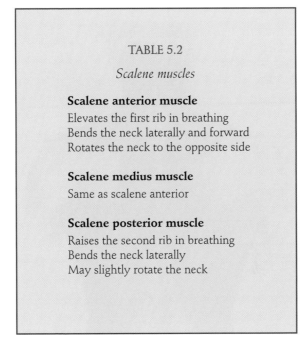

TABLE 5.2

Scalene muscles

Scalene anterior muscle
Elevates the first rib in breathing
Bends the neck laterally and forward
Rotates the neck to the opposite side

Scalene medius muscle
Same as scalene anterior

Scalene posterior muscle
Raises the second rib in breathing
Bends the neck laterally
May slightly rotate the neck

TREATMENT OPTIONS

Traditional treatment options include the following:

- Weight loss, postural re-education, shoulder muscle exercises
- Physical modalities for pain relief (heat, cold, electrical stimulation, ultrasound)
- Spinal manipulation
- Manual release and/or injection of scalene MTrPs
- Surgical removal of the first rib
- Surgical removal of one of the scalene muscles.

As with piriformis syndrome, it is reasonable to consider botulinum toxin treatment for thoracic outlet syndrome resulting from scalene muscle tension or enlargement caused by MTrPs. However, special precautions should be considered when injecting the scalene muscles because of the possibility of weakening these primary muscle(s) of respiration (Simons et al, 1999), the potential for pneumothorax, and the

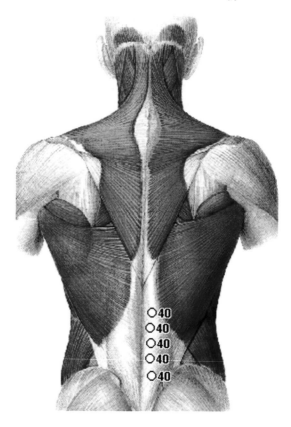

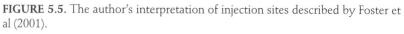

FIGURE 5.5. The author's interpretation of injection sites described by Foster et al (2001).

close proximity to vascular/nerve structures. For these reasons, special imaging techniques (CT, fluoroscopy, ultrasound) most likely are warranted. Effective and safe injection of these muscles takes considerable skill and a thorough working knowledge of the anatomy of that region.

LOW BACK PAIN

Because back pain has a lifetime prevalence of about 90%, there exists a profound rationale for recognizing the cause of and developing new and effective treatments for this symptom. A significant number of cases do not resolve with general medical treatment within 5 weeks and subsequently become chronic. The pharmacoeconomic impact of chronic back pain in the United States suggests a cost of 50 billion US$ each year. Agents commonly used for chronic low back pain include nonsteroidal anti-inflammatory agents (NSAIDS), spasmolytics, antidepressants, muscle relaxants, and opioids. Since intramuscular injections of BTX-A have proven safe and effective in relieving pain in focal dystonia, effects of BTX-A in chronic low back pain sufferers were evaluated in the following double-blind, prospective study (Foster et al, 2001) of 31 chronic back pain sufferers:

- SELECTION CRITERIA

  Low back pain (between lumbar 1 and sacral 1) for no less than 6 months and with pain lateralization. The majority of the patients had no clear idea as to the cause of their pain. All patients were on a variety of medications and were advised NOT to discontinue treatment.

- EXCLUSION CRITERIA

  Pain duration of less than 6 months, age less than 18 years, presence of systemic inflammatory disorder, acute pathology (confirmed by MRI), allergy /sensitivity to BTX-A, injection of anesthetics/corticosteroids to the lumbosacral spine within 12 weeks.

- TREATMENT

  Patients received an intramuscular injection of either 0.4 mL of BTX-A reconstituted to 100 U/mL in preservative-free 0.9% saline or 0.4 mL saline (vehicle) in each of five lumbar or lumbosacral sites (Figure 5.5).

- RESULTS

  Results were recorded at baseline, at 3 weeks (VAS), and at 8 weeks (VAS and OLBPQ) post treatment using two scoring devices:
  - *Visual Analogue Scale (VAS):* a 10-cm horizontal line with the extremes labeled No Pain and Worst Back Pain. Patients mark a point corresponding to the perceived pain; its distance from the No Pain point is measured. Significant response: Scores improved by 50%.

TABLE 5.3

Patient demographics[1]

Patients	BTX-A	Placebo (saline)
Sample size	16 (8/8)	15 (7/8)
Mean age (range, yrs.)	47.0 (20–73)	46.4 (21–65)
Mean pain (duration, yrs.)	5.7 (0.5–20)	8.1 (1–30)
Presenting tender points	12 (L-1–S-1)	11 (L-2–S-1)
Presenting trigger points	1	2
With spasms	2 (1 during injection)	2 (2 during injection)
Disc disease history		
L-5–S-1 (had surgery)	2 (1)	4 (2)
Had neurologic deficits	2	3

Results[1]

	VAS (3 wks)	VAS (8 wks)	OLBPQ (8 wks)
BTX-A	Some relief: 13/15 (86%) Improved by >50%: 11/15 (73.3%)	Improved by >50%: 9/15 (60%)	Functional improvement in 10/15 (66.7%)
Vehicle (saline)	Some relief: 5/16 (31%) Improved by >50%: 4/16 (25%)	Improved by >50%: 2/16 (12.5%)	Functional improvement in 3/14 (18.8%)
Difference	$P = 0.012$; 48% (95% CI, 11.7–80.1%)	$P = 0.009$; 47.5% (95% CI, 10.5–79.1%)	$P = 0.011$; 47.9% (95% CI, 10.9–79.9%)

CI, confidence interval.
[1]*Foster et al, 2001.*

- *Oswestry Low Back Pain Questionnaire (OLBPQ):* scores pain and functional ability in nine subsets of activities (personal care, lifting, walking, sitting, standing, sleeping, sex, social life, and traveling). Functional improvement: improvement of ≥ 2 (40%) in pain plus at least 1 subset.

Results (Table 5.3) indicate that compared with vehicle alone (saline injections), intramuscular BTX-A resulted in significantly greater clinical improvement in low back pain using the methods described.

The possibility that overactive paraspinal musculature and/or MTrPs (Dejung, 1999) may contribute to low back pain provides a rationale for the use of BTX-A, which reduces muscular tone by blocking release of ACh at motor nerve endings. As discussed in Chapter 2, motor nerve blockade need not be the only mechanism by which BTX-A induces relief from back pain. As discussed by Foster et al, in addition to reduction of muscle spasm, BTX-A may also produce a number of clinically important effects. Such effects might include reduction of intrafusal spindle activity, impairment of sympathetic transmission involved in spinal pathways involved in low back pain, and direct analgesic activity by reduction of nociceptive neurons or their metabolites.

REFERENCES

Beatty RA. The piriformis muscle syndrome: A simple diagnostic maneuver. *Neurosurgery* 34:512–4, 1994.

Brückle W, Suckfull M, Fleckenstein W, Weiss C, Müller W. [Tissue pO_2 measurement in taut back musculature (m. erector spinae)]. [German]. *Zeitschrift fur Rheumatologie* 49:208–216, 1990.

Cazzato G and Walton JN. The pathology of the muscle spindle. A study of biopsy material in various muscular and neuromuscular diseases. *J Neurol Sci* 7:15–70, 1968.

Chen WS. Sciatica due to piriformis pyomyositis. Report of a case. *J Bone Joint Surg Am* 74:1546–1548, 1992.

Chen WS, Wan YL. Sciatica caused by piriformis muscle syndrome: Report of two cases. *J Formos Med Assoc* 91:647–650, 1992.

Cheshire WP, Abashian SW, Mann JD. Botulinum toxin in the treatment of myofascial pain syndrome. *Pain* 59:65–69, 1994.

Childers MK. Rationale for injection procedures for botulinum toxin type A in skeletal limb muscles. *Eur J Neurol* 4(suppl 2):37–40, 1997.

Childers MK, Kornegay JN, Aoki R, Ottaviani L, Bogan DJ, Petroski G. Evaluating motor endplate-targeted injections of botulinum toxin type A in a canine model. *Muscle Nerve* 21:653–655,1998.

Childers MK, Wilson DJ, Gnatz SM, Conway RR, Sherman AK. Botulinum toxin type A use in piriformis muscle syndrome: A pilot study. *Am J Phys Med Rehabil,* in press.

Couppe C, Midttun A, Hilden J, Jorgensen U. Spontaneous needle electromyographic activity in myofascial trigger points in the infraspinatus muscle: A blinded assessment. *J Musculoskeletal Pain* 9(3):7–17, 2001.

DeBassio WA, Schnitzler RM, Parsons RL. Influence of lanthanum on transmitter release at the neuromuscular junction. *J Neurobiol* 2:263–278, 1971.

Dejung B. Die Behandlung unspezifischer chronischer Rückenschmerzen mit manueller Triggerpunkt-Therapie [Treatment of chronic low back pain with manual trigger point therapy]. *Manuelle Medizin* 37:124–131, 1999.

Dobrusin R. An osteopathic approach to conservative management of thoracic outlet syndromes. [Review]. *J Am Osteopath Assoc* 89:1046–1050, 1989.

de Paiva A, Meunier FA, Molgo J, Aoki KR, Dolly JO. Functional repair of motor endplates after botulinum neurotoxin type A poisoning: Biphasic switch of synaptic activity between nerve sprouts and their parent terminals. *Proc Natl Acad Sci USA* 96:3200–3205, 1999.

Fishman LM, Zybert PA. Electrophysiologic evidence of piriformis syndrome. *Arch Phys Med Rehabil* 73:359–364, 1992.

Foster L, Clapp L, Erickson M, Jabbari B. Botulinum toxin A and chronic low back pain: A randomized, double-blind study. *Neurology* 56:1290–1293, 2001.

Fricton JR, Auvinen MD, Dykstra D, Schiffman E. Myofascial pain syndrome: Electromyographic changes associated with local twitch response. *Arch Phys Med Rehabil* 66:314–317, 1985.

Fricton JR. Myofascial pain syndrome. [Review]. *Neurol Clin* 7:413–427, 1989.

Hallin RP. Sciatic pain and the piriformis muscle. *Postgrad Med* 74:69–72, 1983.

Heuser J and Miledi R. Effects of lanthanum ions on function and structure of frog neuromuscular junctions. *Proc R Soc Lond B Biol Sci* 179:247–260, 1971.

Hong CZ. Persistence of local twitch response with loss of conduction to and from the spinal cord. *Arch Phys Med Rehabil* 75:12–16, 1994.

Hong CZ, Simons DG. Histological findings of responsive loci in a myofascial trigger spot of rabbit skeletal muscle from where localized twitch responses could be elicited [abstract]. *Arch Phys Med Rehabil* 77:962, 1996.

Hong CZ, Simons DG. Pathophysiologic and electrophysiologic mechanisms of myofascial trigger points. [Review]. *Arch Phys Med Rehabil* 79:863–872, 1998.

Hong CZ, Torigoe Y. Electrophysiological characteristics of localized twitch responses in responsive taut bands of rabbit skeletal muscle. *J Musculoskeletal Pain* 2:17–43, 1994.

Hong CZ, Torigoe Y. Electrophysiological characteristics of localized twitch responses in responsive taut bands of rabbit skeletal muscle. *J Musculoskeletal Pain* 1:15–34, 1995.

Hong CZ, Yu J. Spontaneous electrical activity of rabbit trigger spot after transection of *Spinal Cord* and peripheral nerve. *J Musculoskeletal Pain* 6:45–58, 1998.

Hubbard DR, Berkoff GM. Myofascial trigger points show spontaneous needle EMG activity. *Spine* 18:1803–1807, 1993.

Ito Y, Miledi R, Vincent A. Transmitter release induced by a 'factor' in rabbit serum. *Proc R Soc Lond B Biol Sci* 187:235–241, 1974.

Jankiewicz JJ, Hennrikus WL, Houkom JA. The appearance of the piriformis muscle syndrome in computed tomography and magnetic resonance imaging. A case report and review of the literature. [Review]. *Clin Orthop Rel Res* 205–209, 1991.

Jankovic J, Brin MF. Therapeutic uses of botulinum toxin. [Review]. *N Engl J Med* 324:1186–1194, 1991.

Julsrud ME. Piriformis syndrome. *J Am Podiatr Med Assoc* 79:128–131, 1989.

Kao JT, Woolson ST. Piriformis tendon repair failure after total hip replacement. *Orthop Rev* 21:171–174, 1992.

Kimura J. Electrodiagnosis in diseases of nerve and muscle: *Principles and practice.* Philadelphia: FA Davis, 1989, p. 631.

Kinahan AM, Douglas MJ. Piriformis pyomyositis mimicking epidural abscess in a parturient. *Can J Anaesth* 42:240–245, 1995.

Ku A, Kern H, Lachman E, Nagler W. Sciatic nerve impingement from piriformis hematoma due to prolonged labor [letter]. *Muscle Nerve* 18:789–790, 1995.

LaBan MM, Meerschaert JR, Taylor RS. Electromyographic evidence of inferior gluteal nerve compromise: An early representation of recurrent colorectal carcinoma. *Arch Phys Med Rehabil* 63:33–35, 1982.

Liley AW. An investigation of spontaneous activity at the neuromuscular junction of the rat. *J Physiol (Lond)* 132:650–666, 1956.

Lu MY, Dong BJ, Ma XY. [Piriformis syndrome and its operative treatment: an analysis of sixty cases]. [Chinese]. *Chung-Hua Wai Ko Tsa Chih [Chinese Journal of Surgery]* 23:483–4, 510, 1985.

Mense S, Simons DG, Russell IJ. *Muscle pain: Understanding its nature, diagnosis, and treatment.* Lippincott Williams & Wilkins, Philadelphia, 2001.

Noftal F. The piriformis syndrome. *Can J Surg* 31:210–210, 1988.

Pang D and Wessel HB. Thoracic outlet syndrome. [Review]. *Neurosurgery* 22:105–121, 1988.

Parziale JR, Hudgins TH, Fishman LM. The piriformis syndrome. [Review]. *Am J Orthop* 25:819–823, 1996.

Reitinger A, Radner H, Tilscher H, Hanna M, Windisch A, Feigl W. Morphologische Untersuchung an Triggerpunkten [Morphologic study of trigger points]. *Manuelle Medizin* 34:256–262, 1996.

Sayson SC, Ducey JP, Maybrey JB, Wesley RL, Vermilion D. Sciatic entrapment neuropathy associated with an anomalous piriformis muscle. *Pain* 59:149–152, 1994.

Simons DG. Do endplate noise and spikes arise from normal motor endplates? *Am J Phys Med Rehabil* 80(2):134–140, 2001.

Simons DG, Hong C-Z, Simons LS. Endplate potentials are common to midfiber myofacial trigger points [original should be myofascial]. *Am J Phys Med Rehabil* 81(3):212–222, March 2002.

Simons DG, Stolov WC. Microscopic features and transient contraction of palpable bands in canine muscle. *Am J Phys Med* 55:65–88, 1976.

Simons DG, Travell JG. Myofascial origins of low back pain. 1. Principles of diagnosis and treatment. *Postgrad Med* 73:66–70, 1983a.

Simons DG, Travell JG. Myofascial origins of low back pain. 2. Torso muscles. *Postgrad Med* 73:81–92, 1983b.

Simons DG, Travell JG. Myofascial origins of low back pain. 3. Pelvic and lower extremity muscles. *Postgrad Med* 73:99–105, 1983c.

Simons DG, Travell JG, Simons LS. *Travell & Simons' myofascial pain and dysfunction: The trigger point manual,* vol. 1, ed. 2. Baltimore: Williams & Wilkins, 1999.

Solheim LF, Siewers P, Paus B. The piriformis muscle syndrome. Sciatic nerve entrapment treated with section of the piriformis muscle. *Acta Orthop Scand* 52:73–75, 1981.

Steiner C, Staubs C, Ganon M, Buhlinger C. Piriformis syndrome: Pathogenesis, diagnosis, and treatment. *J Am Osteopath Assoc* 87:318–323, 1987.

Sucher BM. Thoracic outlet syndrome: A myofascial variant: Part 2. Treatment. [Review]. *J Am Osteopath Assoc* 90:810–812, 1990.

Travell JG, Simons DG. *Myofascial pain and dysfunction: The trigger point manual,* vol 2. Williams & Wilkins, Baltimore, 1992.

Urschel HCJ. Management of the thoracic-outlet syndrome. [Review]. *N Engl J Med* 286:1140–1143, 1972.

Wheeler AH, Goolkasian P, Gretz SS. A randomized, double-blind, prospective pilot study of botulinum toxin injection for refractory, unilateral, cervicothoracic, paraspinal, myofascial pain syndrome. *Spine* 23:1662–1666, 1998.

Wiederholt WC. "End-plate noise" in electromyography. *Neurology* 20:214–224, 1970.

Windisch A, Reitinger A, Traxler H, et al. Morphology and histochemistry of myogelosis. *Clin Anat* 12:266–271, 1999.

CHAPTER SIX

Martin K. Childers

PAIN AND DISORDERED MOTOR CONTROL

THE IDEA BEHIND THE USE OF BOTULINUM TOXIN TYPE A (BTX-A) FOR SOME painful conditions is that pain relief may result not only from local muscle paralysis and peripheral antinociception but also from a decrease in the reflex muscle tone. This chapter discusses the potential benefits of decreasing reflex muscle tone from a clinical perspective.

MUSCLE SPINDLES

Muscle spindles are special sensory structures called mechanoreceptors that respond to physical changes in muscle length. Muscle spindles are made of small, spindle-shaped muscle fibers called intrafusal muscle fibers, named for their location within ordinary "extrafusal" skeletal muscle fibers. The spindles are clustered in small bundles surrounded by a protective fluid-filled capsule and lie in parallel with extrafusal fibers. Figure 6.1 shows a micrograph of a muscle spindle.

Muscle spindles may be thought of as space-saving devices. Using information from the spindle, the spinal cord can help regulate muscle tension and position without having to transmit information all the

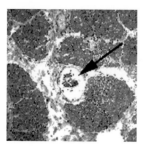

FIGURE 6.1. Micrograph from skeletal muscle, transverse 10µ cryosection. *Arrow* points to a muscle spindle. Note the clear area (fluid-filled capsule) that surrounds the spindle. Stain: H&E. Magnification: 20X. (*Source:* author.)

way to the brain. The ends of the muscle spindles are connected to tendon, connective tissue, or extrafusal muscle fibers. When the entire muscle is stretched, tension is placed on the spindle apparatus. Since the muscle spindle is also connected to sensory nerve endings, called 1a afferents, stretching results in activation of the spindle sensory endings. The sensory component (found in the middle part of the spindle) responds to changes in muscle length.

Once the spinal cord receives information that the spindles have been stretched, a special motor neuron, the gamma motor neuron (relaying signals from the spinal cord to the ends of the spindle) causes the muscle spindle to contract, and subsequently "resets" the sensory nerve. In a way, the gamma motor neuron acts like a thermostat to control how sensitive the sensory structure is to changes in the length of the muscle.

The Relation of Muscle Spindles to Painful Conditions

There appears to be little evidence that painful muscle areas, such as trigger points, are associated with a structural change or sensory structure such as the muscle spindle. However, in certain conditions of abnormal muscle activity, the spindle is intimately involved. In the spastic condition, for example, the stretch reflex is enhanced for a variety of reasons, such as a lack of inhibition from spinal cord interneurons. Whatever the reason, muscle spindle physiology in the spastic condition is an important regulator of muscle tone.

Pain is often associated with spasticity, and this topic is explored in detail below. While not clearly understood, or rigorously tested, an association can be made between abnormal spindle physiology and painful muscular conditions or "muscle spasms." It has been the author's clinical observation that BTX-A at doses lower than anticipated for relief of hypertonia are effective for the relief of pain associated with spasticity or dystonia. One could speculate that these lower doses may be enough to effectively weaken or "reset" the intrinsic (spindle) fibers, and thus indirectly result in pain relief.

Therefore, the idea behind the use of BTX-A for some painful conditions is that pain relief may result not only from local muscle paralysis but from a decrease in the reflex muscle tone.

Implications of BTX-A as a Modifier of Spindle Discharge

While there is yet to be definitive evidence based on humans, if BTX-A does modify spindle discharge, then painful muscle syndromes that are regulated by spindle physiology might be effectively treated through local injections. Experiments in rats have shown that BTX-A reduces spindle discharge, probably by altering the sensitivity of spindle physiology. As a result of such altered physiology, BTX-A may cause changes in the way muscles are activated either by volitional control or by altering an abnormal central programming.

Also, there is evidence suggesting that treatments that increase spindle activity may enhance uptake of BTX-A into muscles. In an experiment by Hesse et al, 10 patients with lower limb spasticity were treated with BTX-A injections and evaluated by computer gait analysis and clinical measures of muscle tone. The difference between the two groups was that one group received electrical stimulation to muscles of the lower leg six times each day for 3 days after BTX-A injection while the other group received only injections. Results showed superior improvement in the group of patients receiving electrical stimulation compared with the group receiving injections alone.

Electrical stimulation causes muscles to contract, and effectively stretches muscle fibers. One example of the use of electrical stimulation can be seen in patients with spinal paralysis. Patients with complete paralysis from spinal cord injury can actually maintain their muscle mass by using electrical stimulation regularly. Another example can be seen in the use of electrical stimulation in rehabilitation of athletes following knee surgery. Electrical stimulation might be similarly effective when used in combination with BTX-A for painful muscle syndromes.

Since muscle spindles are protected by a thick, fluid-filled capsule, uptake of BTX-A in spindles likely occurs by a specific acceptor. Rosales et al (1996) demonstrated increased vulnerability to the effects of BTX-A in spindle endings which contained bag 1 fibers (spindles contain nerve endings of three types, termed bag 1, bag 2, and chain). The important point here is that bag 1 endings are most active during dynamic (active) stretching. Theoretically, treatments such as electrical stimulation or active stretching activities might enhance the clinical effects of BTX-A injections in painful syndromes.

Muscle Spindles and Static Stretching

The author has occasionally prescribed a modality known as "inhibitory casting" following BTX-A treatment for severe spasticity, the idea being that cast application provides low-load, long-duration stretch on spastic muscles, and thus alters the activity of the spindle for a finite time. One way in which spindle activity is supposedly measured is by performing an electrophysiologic test known as "vibratory inhibition of the H reflex." The author's research measuring H reflex inhibition during casting lends support to the idea that during application of an inhibitory cast, motor neuron excitability (probably mediated by the spindle) is decreased in the spastic upper limb.

Other related research also supports this theory by demonstrating alpha motor neuron reflex inhibition following application of circumferential pressure in subjects with spinal cord injury. Thus, some treatments that involve static stretching (versus dynamic or active stretching), when performed during the first few hours of administration of BTX-A, might paradoxically inhibit the desirable paralytic effects of the toxin. Although these studies tend to support the use of static stretching in the spastic condition, timing with BTX-A administration may be important. While more research is needed to establish the usefulness and timing of casting (or static stretching) in combination with the treatment of spasticity and painful muscle conditions, this modality might be useful as an adjunctive therapy when prescribed a few days after initial injection.

SPASTICITY

Spasticity is a term given to describe a condition associated with abnormal muscle tone due to an abnormality of the central nervous system. Specifically, spasticity is considered to be a hallmark of an upper motor neuron syndrome (as opposed to a lower motor neuron syndrome). Features of the upper motor neuron syndrome include

- spasticity
- clonus
- increased reflexes
- weakness
- lack of dexterity
- slowness in the initiation of movement.

If a patient presents with abnormal muscle tone and findings which are *not* consistent with an upper motor neuron syndrome, spasticity would not be considered the appropriate term to describe the condition. In fact, while some physiology literature uses the terms *spasticity* and *dystonia* interchangeably, from a clinical standpoint dystonia refers to a type of disorder of movement that usually is *not* seen within the context of an upper motor neuron syndrome. As would be expected, treatment of dystonia is quite different from the treatment of spasticity.

Spasticity may be manifested in the patient as abnormal resistance to movement. For example, when the patient's gamma motor neuron is overly sensitive to stretch tension ("gamma" spasticity), on examination the faster you attempt to move the spastic limb, the more resistance you encounter. This is termed "velocity-dependent" muscle resistance. In addition to observing velocity-dependent muscle resistance, you should see signs of the upper motor neuron syndrome (brisk reflexes, weakness, and lack of dexterity). Spasticity is not seen in patients with normal central nervous system physiology, and should not be confused with "muscle spasm."

Muscle spasm is not a specifically defined medical term, and generally refers to pain associated with muscle injury or is used in the context of a myofascial pain syndrome. Most people are familiar with a back muscle "spasm" or muscle "cramp." These involuntary contractions of individual muscles or groups of muscles may come on suddenly, without warning, and be excruciatingly painful. Muscle spasm may be related to irritability of the muscle spindle or due to a temporary electrolyte imbalance (as is seen after vigorous athletic training). The important point is that while muscle spasms are not related to spasticity per se, muscle spasms may occur in patients with spasticity. Pain associated with spasticity may be related to muscle spasm—not necessarily to the increased muscle tone that results from a problem in the central nervous system.

Antispastic Agents and Pain Relief

This is a complex topic. Simply stated, agents that either decrease motor neuron excitability or increase the inhibitory influence on the alpha motor neuron will reduce muscle tone, and thus might also reduce pain associated with muscular hyperactivity.

Some antispastic agents work by increasing the inhibitory influence of the amino acid gamma-aminobutyric acid (GABA), which, in turn, activates either (a) chloride channels (hyperpolarizing the postsynaptic membrane making it "harder" to depolarize) or (b) cyclic adenosine monophosphate (cAMP), which decreases intracellular calcium ions required for muscle contraction.

The antispastic agent *dantrolene sodium* acts directly on the muscle contractile mechanism by decreasing the availability of intracellular calcium.

Other agents, *tizanadine* and *clonidine* (alpha-2 adrenergic agonists), presumably act by mechanisms that increase noradrenergic inhibition to reduce motor neuron excitability.

BTX-A as Therapy for Spasticity

BTX-A may work in (gamma) spasticity by peripheral mechanisms rather than by central mechanisms of increasing inhibition. In patients with hemiplegic spasticity, for example, BTX-A injections into spastic calf muscles presumably act by focally weakening extrafusal muscle fibers. The functional result in improved walking ability occurs by allowing the spastic leg to roll over the ankle with less resistance to abnormal spastic contractions.

There is indirect evidence to suggest that BTX-A might also have an even greater paralytic effect on the intrafusal fibers of muscle spindle compared with extrafusal fibers in spastic patients. This property of greater paralytic effect on the spindle fibers may be useful to the clinician in the treatment of spasticity. If weakening the muscle spindle fibers in the patient with spasticity would decrease the spindle afferent discharge, then a reduced hyperactive stretch reflex should be observed in spastic patients. This putative property of BTX-A is particularly desirable in the setting of a patient with hemiplegic gait with ankle clonus.

Clinical Evidence in Spasticity Literature

There is evidence that the paralytic properties of BTX-A are enhanced in patients given electrical stimulation to spastic muscles during the first few days after injection with botulinum toxin. Some experts speculate that the enhanced activity of BTX-A is due to increased spindle discharge from electrical stimulation.

BTX-A might also be useful to the clinician in the treatment of patients with spasticity accompanied by painful spasms. For while oral antispastic agents also may be helpful in reducing the pain related to spasticity and muscle spasms, many patients cannot tolerate side effects of these agents (eg, sedation, weakness). It is the author's experience that doses of botulinum toxin even lower than those required to reduce spasticity have analgesic effects when injected into painful muscles. This experience is also reported in the spasticity literature.

Also, the author believes that information gained from spasticity cases might be applicable to patients with myofascial pain, as similar mechanisms may contribute to painful spasms whether due to spasticity or other reasons. While controversial, the trigger point (seen in myofascial pain syndromes) may be associated with abnormal spindle function. In this scenario, overactive spindle mechanisms might respond effectively to local injections of BTX-A, resulting in decreased outflow to extrafusal fibers and subsequent diminished spasm.

DYSTONIA

Dystonia is a condition that causes involuntary muscular contraction, often resulting in bizarre twisting postures. It was first termed "dystonia musculorum deformans" by Oppenheim to describe the progressive nature of the twisting movements that often led to deforming postures.

The most common cause of dystonia is idiopathic, with or without a hereditary pattern. Other causes include head trauma, peripheral injury, stroke and encephalitis. Focal dystonias affect only one segment or area of the body. Most of us are familiar with focal dystonia of the neck muscles, which causes rotation (torticollis). Other forms of focal dystonia include involuntary eye closing (blepharospasm), writer's cramp, and spastic speech (spasmotic dysphonia).

Dystonia and Pain

Some investigators have reported that as many as 70% of patients with some forms of cervical dystonia have pain associated with involuntary muscle contraction. Other forms of focal dystonias are also associated with pain that is thought to arise from involuntary contraction of muscles. However, it is beyond the scope of this work to adequately describe the nature, diagnosis, and treatment of dystonia. The reader is urged to read one of several excellent resources on the topic listed in the bibliography at the end of this chapter and in the Appendix. Clearly, there appears to be a close relationship between focal dystonia and pain; in fact, the FDA has licensed the use of BTX-A for this very indication.

Diagnosis

Typically, neurologists with special training and interests in movement disorders treat the dystonias. Since most dystonias are diagnosed by clinical evaluation, it is important that any patient considered to have an undiagnosed dystonia be evaluated by a specialist with experience and training in movement disorders.

To find a movement disorder specialist in your area, contact

Dystonia Medical Research Foundation
One East Wacker Drive, Suite 2430
Chicago, IL 60601-1905 USA
800-377-3978, or 312-755-0198

Treatment

There is no single agent (systemic or local) that is uniformly effective in the treatment of all dystonias. Many movement disorder experts feel that local injections of botulinum toxin are the treatment of choice for focal dystonias.

Before determining treatment, however, one must confirm a diagnosis of focal dystonia as opposed to a myofascial pain syndrome. Most dystonias result in twisting postures, are worse with voluntary movement or stress, and are insidious in onset. However, the author has seen a few patients with involuntary muscular contractions of the trapezius, levator scapulae, and various shoulder girdle muscles that did *not* result in the stereotypical dystonic limb postures, but *did* present with pain, muscle hypertrophy, frustration with prior (ineffective) medical treatment for the relief of pain, and involuntary muscle contractions found on electromyography (EMG) exam.

EMG may be helpful in distinguishing pain arising from muscular "spasm" from pain arising from the involuntary muscular contractions associated with dystonia. Pain associated with the latter may be managed most effectively with local injections of botulinum toxin, whereas the former may be amenable to other treatment. Consider a consultation with a neurologist or physiatrist for EMG in these cases.

Other research has shown that abnormal muscle contractions seen in dystonia can be modified by blocking afferent nerves (signals going from the spinal cord toward the muscle) with local injections of lidocaine. Patients with dystonia often learn to take advantage of "sensory tricks" that similarly alter abnormal muscle activity.

In summary, the idea behind the use of BTX-A for some painful conditions is that pain relief may result not only from local muscle paralysis but from a decrease in the reflex muscle tone.

REFERENCES

Botte MJ, Abrams RA, Bodine-Fowler SC. Treatment of acquired muscle spasticity using phenol peripheral nerve blocks. [Review]. *Orthopedics* 18:151–159,1995.

Brin MF, Fahn S, Moskowitz C, et al. Localized injections of botulinum toxin for the treatment of focal dystonia and hemifacial spasm. *Adv Neurol* 50:599–608, 1988.

Calne S. Local treatment of dystonia and spasticity with injections of botulinum-A toxin. *Axone* 14:85–88, 1993.

Davidoff RA. Antispasticity drugs: Mechanisms of action. [Review]. *Ann Neurol* 17:107–116, 1985.

Grandas F. Clinical application of botulinum toxin. [Review] [Spanish]. *Neurologia* 10:224–233, 1995.

Herman R. The myotatic reflex. Clinico-physiological aspects of spasticity and contracture. *Brain* 93:273–312, 1970.

Hesse S, Jahnke MT, Luecke D, Mauritz KH. Short-term electrical stimulation enhances the effectiveness of botulinum toxin in the treatment of lower limb spasticity in hemiparetic patients. *Neurosci Lett* 201:37–40, 1995.

Hesse S, Krajnik J, Luecke D, Jahnke MT, Gregoric M, Mauritz KH. Ankle muscle activity before and after botulinum toxin therapy for lower limb extensor spasticity in chronic hemiparetic patients. *Stroke* 27:455–460, 1996.

Hesse S, Lucke D, Malezic M, et al. Botulinum toxin treatment for lower limb extensor spasticity in chronic hemiparetic patients. *J Neurol Neurosurg Psychiatry* 57:1321–1324, 1994.

Hong CZ, Hsueh TC. Difference in pain relief after trigger point injections in myofascial pain patients with and without fibromyalgia [see Comments]. *Arch Phys Med Rehabil* 77:1161–1166, 1996.

Hong CZ, Simons DG. Pathophysiologic and electrophysiologic mechanisms of myofascial trigger points. [Review]. *Arch Phys Med Rehabil* 79:863–872, 1998.

Hughes AJ. Botulinum toxin in clinical practice. [Review]. *Drugs* 48:888–893, 1994.

Jankovic J, Schwartz K, Donovan DT. Botulinum toxin treatment of cranial-cervical dystonia, spasmodic dysphonia, other focal dystonias and hemifacial spasm. *J Neurol Neurosurg Psychiatry* 53:633–639, 1990.

Lagueny A, Burbaud P. Mechanism of action, clinical indication and results of treatment of botulinum toxin. [Review] [French]. *Neurophysiol Clin* 26:216–226, 1996.

Pacchetti C, Albani G, Martignoni E, Godi L, Alfonsi E, Nappi G. "Off" painful dystonia in Parkinson's disease treated with botulinum toxin. *Mov Disord* 10:333–336, 1995.

Price R, Lehmann JF, Boswell-Bessette S, Burleigh A, deLateur BJ. Influence of cryotherapy on spasticity at the human ankle. *Arch Phys Med Rehabil* 74:300–304, 1993.

Priebe MM, Sherwood AM, Thornby JI, Kharas NF, Markowski J. Clinical assessment of spasticity in spinal cord injury: A multidimensional problem. *Arch Phys Med Rehabil* 77:713–716, 1996.

Pullman SL, Greene P, Fahn S, Pedersen SF. Approach to the treatment of limb disorders with botulinum toxin A. Experience with 187 patients. *Arch Neurol* 53:617–624, 1996.

Rosales RL, Arimura K, Takenaga S, Osame M. Extrafusal and intrafusal muscle effects in experimental botulinum toxin-A injection. *Muscle Nerve* 19:488–496, 1996.

Tona JL, Schneck CM. The efficacy of upper extremity inhibitive casting: A single-subject pilot study. *Am J Occup Ther* 47:901–910, 1993.

Yablon SA, Agana BT, Ivanhoe CB, Boake C. Botulinum toxin in severe upper extremity spasticity among patients with traumatic brain injury: An open-labeled trial. *Neurology* 47:939–944, 1996.

Young RR, Delwaide PJ: Drug therapy: Spasticity (Part I). *N Engl J Med* 304:28–33, 1981.

CHAPTER SEVEN

Martin K. Childers

EQUIPMENT AND INJECTION TECHNIQUES

THERAPY WITH BOTULINUM TOXIN TYPE A (BTX-A) SHOULD BE INDIVIDUALIZED for both the patient and the clinician. Equipment needs may be determined by patient needs, clinician's training, and the anatomic target for injection. For example, injections for blepharospasm are usually given by simple subcutaneous injections around the eye, without the use of special equipment. However, injections into the deep compartments of the low back, such as the psoas major muscle compartment, may require the use of special imaging techniques.

The author does not see the need for operating rooms or special procedure (sterile) rooms equipped with monitoring devices for the purpose of intramuscular injections of BTX-A using small-caliber needles. Most patients can be safely treated in an office setting by experienced clinicians.

For most limb muscles, the author recommends use of electromyography (EMG) or motor point stimulation (e-stim) to identify muscles, particularly the smaller muscles in the forearm. For example, a commonly injected finger flexor muscle, the flexor digitorum sublimis (FDS), is nearly impossible to locate without EMG guidance.

For the clinician who is developing his/her skills in identifying specific muscles for injection with botulinum toxin, the use of simple "audio-only" EMG may further enhance the clinician's understanding of functional anatomy and aid in the decision-making on injection localization.

A summary of the special equipment used for various injection sites is presented in the box below. Information on portable audio EMG units and stimulators is found in Appendix B.

As with any procedure in medicine, it will be important for you to get some "hands on" training by an experienced clinician prior to treating patients with BTX-A by injection for the first time. One medical academy has published training guidelines for physicians who use BTX-A to treat neurological disorders. The author strongly encourages attending training seminars and acquiring some one-on-one instruction before proceeding to treat patients with botulinum toxin.

INJECTION LOCATIONS

The electrophysiologic evidence discussed earlier supports an association with abnormal end-plate activity and myofascial trigger points. The author's research in dogs and mice supports injection techniques

---

EQUIPMENT USED FOR VARIOUS INJECTION SITES

Location	Equipment
Face	None required
Neck	Audio EMG, e-stim
Limbs	Audio EMG, e-stim
Easily accessible trigger points	None required
Deep compartment	Fluoroscopy, ultrasound
Muscles of back	CT and/or EMG
Superficial muscles of the trunk	Audio EMG
Flexors of distal finger joints	E-stim

that either localize motor end plates or place the injection needle in close proximity to motor end plates. Since trigger points should lie in the close proximity to motor end plates, the clinician should attempt to target injections toward the zone or distribution of the motor end plates whenever possible. This is the technique the author employs whenever possible. Although it may seem that attempting to localize such small, discrete areas within a large muscle is much like hunting for a needle in a haystack, there are ways in which you can narrow down the likely location of these discrete points.

It has been shown that end plates do not occur randomly scattered throughout skeletal muscle but in groups or "bands" in most cases. The distribution of these locations is relatively well described in humans, and likely coincides with "motor point" maps published elsewhere. Motor points are areas within muscle where small motor nerves terminate and are used to direct locations for phenol or alcohol blocks.

LOCALIZING MOTOR END PLATES

As the practicality of localizing motor end plates may be problematic, the equipment mentioned above is quite useful. To localize motor end plates, you need to use EMG and have some idea where to start searching within a large muscle. In the case of the trigger point, your task should be somewhat simpler, as you should be able to accurately find the trigger point with the tip of your finger.

Next, connect the EMG to a dual-purpose needle electrode and search for the characteristic noise of the motor end plate. In the case where trigger points are not present, you will need to refer to a motor point chart, or review information on motor end-plate zones in Chapter 3 to increase your chances of finding them. Remember that this technique may not be appropriate in all cases, such as when the patient cannot completely relax the muscle and create electrical silence, or in the case of strap muscles (discussed below) where end-plate "zones" don't really apply.

The motor end plate also is home to the neuromuscular junction. Find the motor end plate, and you've localized the neuromuscular junction. For a more detailed description of the characteristic electrophysiologic features of the motor end plate, read Wiederholt's description of the motor end plate. In short, the characteristic features of the motor end plate are as follows:

- a low-voltage increase in the baseline of about 10–40 mV (the audio EMG sounds similar to holding a seashell to your ear);
- it usually accompanies irregularly firing monophasic spike discharges;
- deep pain is described by the patient.

Once one motor end plate has been localized within the target muscle, the author usually does not hunt for others (because of time issues) but rather assumes that he is within the zone or proximity of other motor end plates. Three of four sites are subsequently injected (as illustrated in below) in a pattern that likely coincides with the midpoint of the muscle fibers. This technique has been confirmed experimentally in dogs, but not in humans, and there are practical issues that need to be confirmed by future clinical research.

If there is too much noise from involuntary muscle activity, consider another injection method such as the motor point method or the anatomic method.

MOTOR POINT METHODS

You cannot localize motor end plates (the site of action of botulinum toxin) using EMG unless the patient is able to completely relax the muscle. Some clinicians feel that they can find the motor end plate using electrical stimulation (either with a needle or surface electrode). However, you may not be entirely correct in assuming that motor end plates and motor "points" are one and the same. There is evidence which shows that motor points (localized with a stimulator) in some muscles are actually places in muscle where small motor nerve endings enter into a portion of the muscle, rather than a motor end plate where the chemical (acetylcholine) responsible for muscle contraction is released. However, in other muscles, the motor point overlies the motor end plate. Since the site of action of BTX-A is at the motor end plate, it is important to be able to localize this area within large muscles, but motor points are probably reasonably close and may be a good alternative in some situations. If you want to explore this technique further, the author suggests reviewing studies listed in the references at the end of the chapter and offers the following summary of earlier research examining the association between motor end plates and motor points in muscle biopsies.

- Muscles with Long Fibers Where Motor End Plates Overlie the Motor Point
  - Biceps
  - Deltoid
  - Flexor carpi radialis
  - Flexor digitorum sublimis
  - Vastus internus
  - Sternomastoid
  - Palmaris longus

The association between the motor point and motor end plate is due to the parallel arrangement of long muscle fibers (see dashed lines below) that form a linear innervation band ("X"). This band of motor end plates (an "end-plate zone") crosses the surface of the muscle at its approximate center:

```
----------------------X----------------------
----------------------X----------------------
----------------------X----------------------
----------------------X----------------------
```

- Muscles in Which the Motor Point Overlies the Motor End Plates
  - Tibialis anterior
  - Brachioradialis

In these muscles, the muscle fibers arise from superficial connective tissue and run deep toward a muscle–tendon junction; therefore, the motor end plates underlie the motor point deep to the surface.

- Muscles in Which the Motor Point is Proximal to the Motor End Plates:
  - Gastrocnemius
  - Peroneus longus

In these muscles, the motor point is proximal to the motor end plate because the muscle fibers receive their innervation several inches distal to the motor point. The motor nerve enters these muscles proximally, and runs along the line of tendon insertion, becoming progressively more superficial. For these reasons, the motor point is easily found at a site superficial and proximal to the motor end plates.

- EQUIPMENT FOR MOTOR POINT LOCALIZATION
    - Peripheral nerve stimulator
    - Surface electrodes or single probe stimulator
    - Electrode gel
    - Dual purpose needle electrode

(Surface) Motor Point Localization Technique

Stimulation intensity: 5–10 mA and 0.5-s duration

- Use surface electrode or probe over muscle belly.
- Observe for muscular contraction coincident with stimulation pulse.
- Continue to reduce current until a minimal contraction is seen.
- Repeat until the lowest intensity stimulation causes a muscle contraction over one point overlying the muscle, and mark that point on the skin.

Intramuscular Motor Point Localization Technique

- Repeat procedure above intramuscularly.
- Sterilize skin.
- Attach lead from needle to cathode (black pole).
- Attach anode (red pole) lead to surface electrode near site of needle entry.
- Insert needle through skin at point previously marked
- Turn stimulator on and increase intensity to 3 or 4 mA.
- Reduce stimulation intensity and probe muscle until a contraction can be observed with only 1 mA or less.

E-stim and Stretching

Since there is indirect evidence to support the contention that overactive spindle activity enhances the paralytic property of botulinum toxin, treatments such as electrical stimulation or muscle stretching, which enhance spindle activity, likely would enhance the effects of the toxin.

- E-STIM OR STRETCHING AFTER BTX-A INJECTION WOULD INCLUDE THE FOLLOWING:
    - Active stretching of injected muscles several times each day for 72 h following injection with BTX-A may enhance treatment effects.
    - Electrical stimulation given several times each day for 72 h following injection may also enhance effects.
    - TENS (transcutaneous electrical neuromuscular stimulation) units can easily be programmed to do this.

A sample prescription written for a patient post botulinum toxin is presented in the box below.

TENS Unit

A TENS unit can be used to localize the surface motor point over a muscle quite easily: Attach one surface electrode to the patient's skin and the other electrode to the back of your own hand. Use a little electrode gel or water and gently run your index finger over the surface of the skin overlying the muscle of interest. Adjust the intensity of the TENS unit until you can actually feel the current beneath your finger; then, decrease the stimulus intensity until you no longer can feel any current except for one point on the skin. This point will correspond to the motor point found using the more traditional technique. If you like, you can verify this by increasing the TENS intensity high enough to elicit a muscle contraction over the tip of your finger!

EMG Activity Method

EMG activity method is yet another method to target injections of BTX-A in muscle. In the case of excessive involuntary muscle contraction, such as with dystonia or spasticity, injecting the area of "most active EMG activity" may potentiate effects of botulinum toxin. For example, some clinicians probe within the small muscles of the forearm in a patient with focal dystonia to identify areas that seem to be the most "noisy" on EMG, and subsequently inject these areas. These audio signals are active motor unit potentials and sound like rain on a

[SAMPLE PRESCRIPTION]

POST BOTULINUM TOXIN

PATIENT:
_____

John Smith

DIAGNOSIS:
_____

myofascial pain syndrome, spasticity due to stroke

PHYSICAL THERAPIST:
_____

1. *"Trial of TENS, post BTX-A injection—Apply electrodes over motor points of injected muscles and stimulate six times daily (30 minutes) for three days"*

2. *"Develop and instruct in a supervised home stretching program."*

3. *"Please treat three times per week for two weeks and provide a report of response to treatment."*

tin roof, as opposed to the lower pitched seashell murmur of the motor end plate potentials.

For patients with spasticity, the same scenario often exists. For example, the patient with a very tightly clenched fist (the "fisted hand") may have massive audio EMG discharges from the flexor digitorum sublimus muscle when the examiner attempts to passively stretch the fingers of the fisted hand. In this case, the author would inject into the areas that are "noisiest" with EMG activity (it would be impossible to localize the motor end plate with such excessive background noise.

Anatomic Method

Armed with the knowledge that motor end plates lie at the midpoint of muscle fibers, another injection method involves targeting the midpoint of muscle fibers based on an estimate of where the fibers are arranged within a muscle. This method is based on odds: the greater number of needle sticks and injection sites within a muscle, the more likely you are to infuse the toxin into the site of action within a muscle.

With only a few exceptions, the majority of motor end plates will be found within the greatest bulk of a muscle. Exploiting this anatomic distribution, some clinicians identify the target muscle, draw a grid over the bulkiest portion of the muscle, and penetrate the skin at a number of the sites marked to distribute the toxin over a large area. This technique may be most useful in large, flat muscles like the trapezius, where motor point or end plate localization can be tedious.

Using careful measurements of the location of motor end plates in dog gastrocnemius muscles, the author compared the effectiveness of the anatomic method with that of the motor end plate targeting method. The results were somewhat surprising, for significant differences were found between the two methods in the small canine muscles. The motor end plate targeting method was experimentally superior, and therefore the author recommends using EMG whenever possible.

While further research is needed to establish which method(s) are most desirable, treatment with BTX-A must always be individualized for the needs of the patient and the skills of the clinician.

SUGGESTED INJECTION SITES

In general, injection localization for BTX-A injection might best be decided using a hierarchy of findings. Consider injecting areas that manifest the following features, with greater importance placed on findings at the top of the list:

1. AREAS OF MOST ACTIVE EMG MOTOR UNIT FIRING (CONTINUOUS NOISE OF MOTOR UNIT FIRING). Finding continuously contracting motor units (the alpha motor neuron at its muscle fibers) when the patient is cooperative and voluntarily attempting to relax the muscle(s) of interest may be consistent with dystonia or

alpha rigidity. When the clinician identifies these features, it may be best to inject the most active area of muscle, regardless of whether or not a motor point or motor end plate can be identified.

2. MOTOR END PLATES FOUND IN ANY MUSCLE BY EMG.

3. MOTOR POINTS IN THE FOLLOWING MUSCLES: Biceps, deltoid, flexor carpi, radialis, flexor digitorum sublimus, vastus internus, sternomastoid, palmaris longus, tibialis anterior, and brachioradialis.

4. MYOFASCIAL TRIGGER POINT(S) WITHIN THE TARGET MUSCLE: Since abnormal motor end plates are probably characteristic features of the trigger point, it may be desirable to inject these areas when found within the target muscle.

See Appendix B for information on injection procedures that is available on video and in print.

The following section illustrates the author's injection techniques using BTX-A for commonly encountered painful conditions involving limb and neck muscles. The reader should be aware that the following illustrations are based upon the author's clinical experience rather than upon prospective studies of BTX-A injection procedures. Accordingly, these sites and BTX-A doses are likely to be modified as clinicians gain more experience using BTX-A in painful conditions and as future prospective research defines optimal delivery methods.

There is considerable variation among investigators with regard to preferred injection technique, dosing, and number of sites injected. The following section provides a general guide for determining dosing and injection techniques for a number of muscles commonly treated with botulinum toxin. It is most important to remember, however, that treatment with BTX-A should always be individualized. Every patient is different and circumstances may dictate variation in the technique applied.

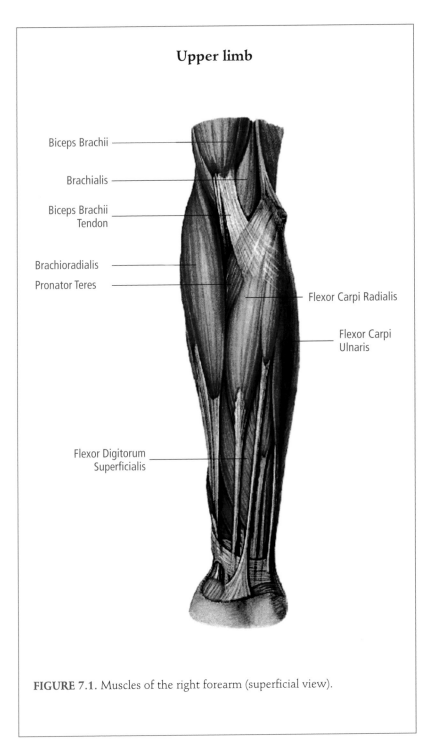

Biceps Brachii

Brachialis

Biceps Brachii
Tendon

Brachioradialis

Pronator Teres

Flexor Carpi Radialis

Flexor Carpi
Ulnaris

Flexor Digitorum
Superficialis

FIGURE 7.1. Muscles of the right forearm (superficial view).

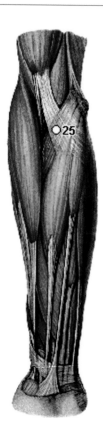

FIGURE 7.2. Suggested injection site for the pronator teres muscle.

INDICATION: Painful excessive pronation of the wrist.

PITFALLS: Overweakening may cause difficulty with daily activities like opening jars.

INJECTION LOCATION: Corresponds to the motor point.

BTX-A DOSE: 25–75 U

DILUTION: 100 mU in 1 cc saline

NUMBER OF SITES: 1

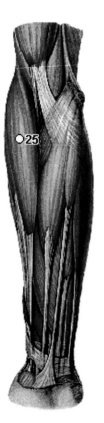

FIGURE 7.3. Suggested injection sites for brachioradialis muscle.

INDICATION: Painful flexion/supination of the elbow. *Note:* This muscle is usually treated in conjunction with the biceps and brachialis muscles.

PITFALLS: Few.

INJECTION LOCATION: Corresponds to motor point.

BTX-A DOSE: 25 U

DILUTION: 100 mU in 1 cc saline

NUMBER OF SITES: 1

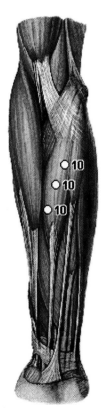

FIGURE 7.4. Suggested injection sites for the flexor digitorum sublimis muscle.

Note: For more detailed information about injection localization for this muscle, see Bickerton et al, 1997).

INDICATION: Painful flexion of the wrist and proximal joints of the fingers.

PITFALLS: Injections proximal to the injection sites shown may miss the muscle fibers.

BTX-A DOSE: 30–100 U

NUMBER OF SITES: 3

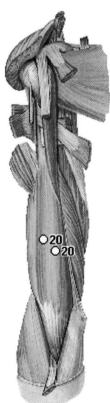

FIGURE 7.5. Suggested injection sites for the brachialis muscle.

Note: This muscle lies deep to the biceps and is an important flexor of the elbow. The author uses a medial injection approach for this muscle.

INDICATION: Painful flexion of the elbow.

PITFALLS: Injections placed superficially will be located in the biceps rather than in the brachialis muscle.

BTX-A DOSE: 30–60 U

NUMBER OF SITES: 2–3

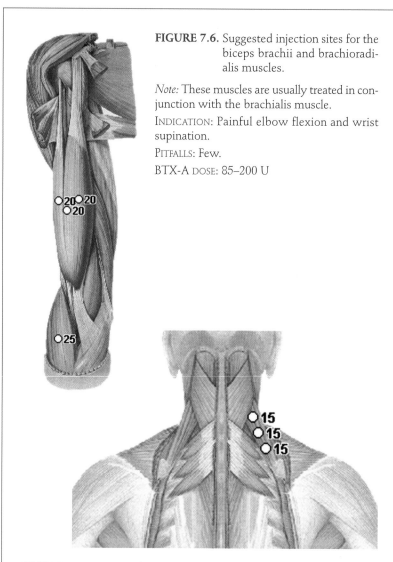

FIGURE 7.6. Suggested injection sites for the biceps brachii and brachioradialis muscles.

Note: These muscles are usually treated in conjunction with the brachialis muscle.

INDICATION: Painful elbow flexion and wrist supination.

PITFALLS: Few.

BTX-A DOSE: 85–200 U

FIGURE 7.7. Suggested injection site for the levator scapula muscle.

ACTION: Elevates scapula.

PITFALLS: If too superficial, injections will be in the trapezius; if too deep, injections will be in paraspinal muscles.

INJECTION LOCATION: As marked.

BTX-A DOSE: 45–75 U

DILUTION: 100 U in 1 cc saline

NUMBER OF SITES: 3

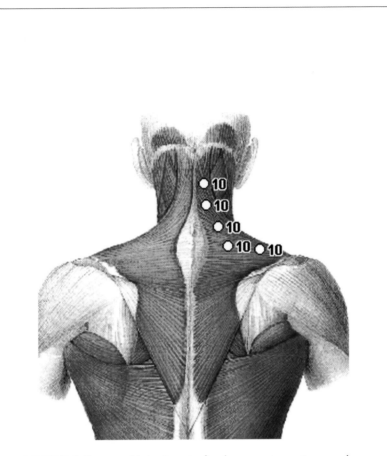

FIGURE 7.8. Suggested injection site for the upper trapezius muscle.

INDICATION: Posterior neck and shoulder pain.

PITFALLS: Few.

BTX-A DOSE: 10–15 U/site (50–100 U total)

DILUTION: 100 U in 1 cc saline

NUMBER OF SITES: 5

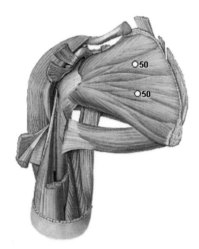

FIGURE 7.9. Suggested injection sites for the subscapularis muscle.

Note: The author uses a medial approach to this muscle using a 50-mm 22-gauge dual-purpose injection needle/electrode (see Appendix A for details). The patient is seated with the involved upper limb extended behind the back to wing the scapula. EMG localization is highly recommended.

INDICATION: Painful internal rotation of the shoulder ("frozen shoulder").

PITFALLS: Injections are located in close proximity to the thorax. The clinician should be wary of inadvertent pleural puncture and pneumothorax as a complication of this procedure.

BTX-A DOSE: 85–200 U

NUMBER OF SITES: 1–2

Lower limb

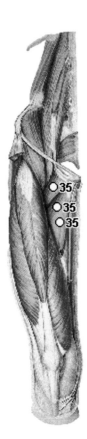

FIGURE 7.10. Suggested injection sites for hip adductor muscles.

Action: Painful adduction of thigh.

Pitfalls: When using electrical stimulation for localization, if the stimulation is too proximal, the needle may contact a branch of the obturator nerve rather than an intramuscular motor point.

Injection location: As marked.

BTX-A dose: 100–200 U

Dilution: 100 U in 3 cc saline

Number of sites: 2–4/muscle

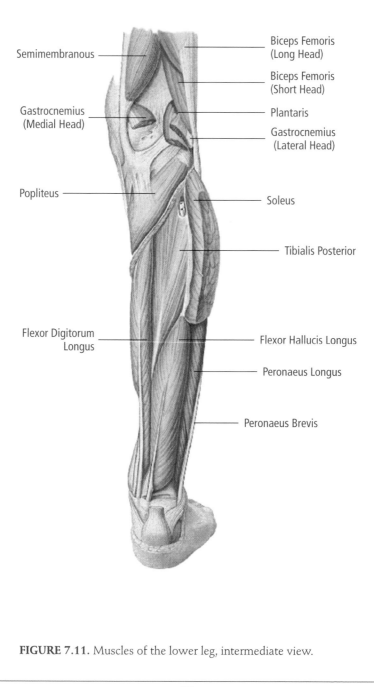

Semimembranous

Biceps Femoris
(Long Head)

Biceps Femoris
(Short Head)

Gastrocnemius
(Medial Head)

Plantaris

Gastrocnemius
(Lateral Head)

Popliteus

Soleus

Tibialis Posterior

Flexor Digitorum
Longus

Flexor Hallucis Longus

Peronaeus Longus

Peronaeus Brevis

FIGURE 7.11. Muscles of the lower leg, intermediate view.

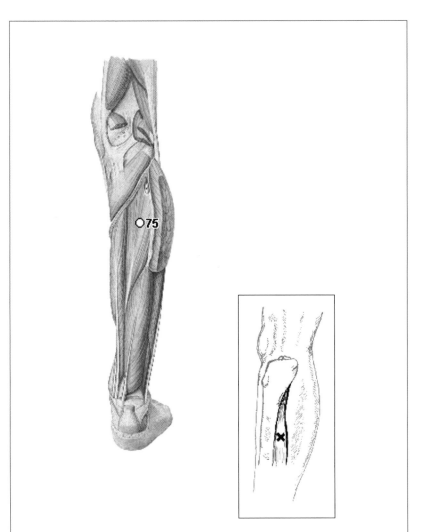

FIGURE 7.12. Suggested injection site of the tibialis posterior muscle.

Note: The author uses an anterior-lateral approach to this muscle *(inset).*

INDICATION: Painful forefoot inversion and plantar flexion.

PITFALLS: Difficult to localize with motor point stimulation; proximity to vessels in posterior compartment of lower limb.

INJECTION LOCATION: As marked.

BTX-A DOSE: 75–100 U

DILUTION: 100 mU in 2 cc saline

NUMBER OF SITES: 1

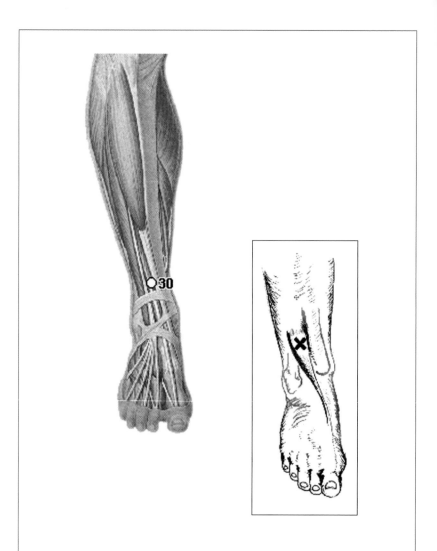

FIGURE 7.13. Suggested injection site for the extensor hallucis longus muscle.

INDICATION: Painful dorsiflexion of the great toe ("hitchhiker's toe").

PITFALLS: Narrow window of needle insertion to hit muscle due to overlying fascia and tendons.

INJECTION LOCATION: As marked.

BTX-A DOSE: 50–75 units

DILUTION: 100 U in 1 cc saline

NUMBER OF SITES: 1

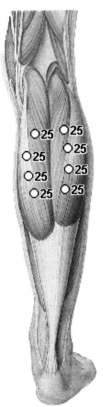

FIGURE 7.14. Suggested injected sites for the gastrocnemius muscles.

Note: This muscle is usually treated in conjunction with the soleus and tibialis posterior muscles.

INDICATION: Painful ankle plantarflexion.

INJECTION LOCATION: As marked.

PITFALLS: Motor point is proximal to end plate zone.

BTX-A DOSE: 100–200 U

DILUTION: 100 U in 3 cc saline

NUMBER OF SITES: 2–4/ muscle

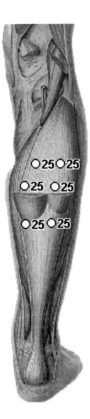

FIGURE 7.15. Suggested injection sites for the soleus muscle.

Note: This muscle is usually treated in conjunction with the gastrocnemius and tibialis posterior muscles.

INDICATION: Painful ankle plantarflexion.

INJECTION LOCATION: As marked.

PITFALLS: This muscle is deep to the gastrocnemius (Figure 7.17). Injections that are too shallow will be in the gastrocnemius rather than in the soleus muscle.

BTX-A DOSE: 100–200 units

DILUTION: 100 U in 3 cc saline

NUMBER OF SITES: 2–4

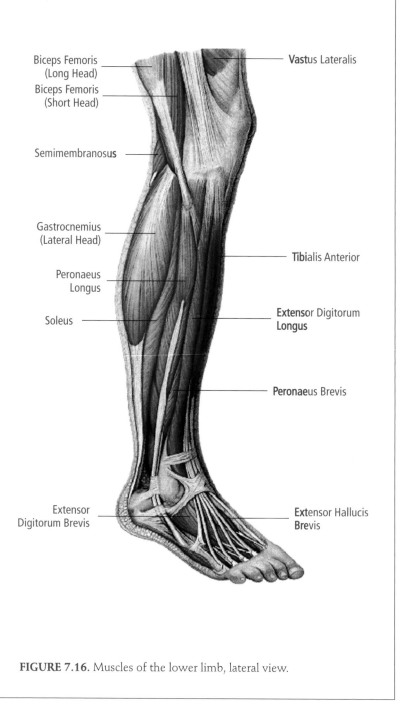

FIGURE 7.16. Muscles of the lower limb, lateral view.

Biceps Femoris (Long Head)

Biceps Femoris (Short Head)

Semimembranosus

Gastrocnemius (Lateral Head)

Peronaeus Longus

Soleus

Extensor Digitorum Brevis

Vastus Lateralis

Tibialis Anterior

Extensor Digitorum **Longus**

Peronaeus Brevis

Extensor Hallucis **Bre**vis

Back

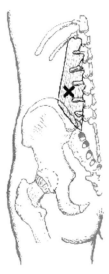

FIGURE 7.17. Suggested injection site for the quadratus lumborum muscle.

INDICATION: Painful lateral trunk flexion.

INJECTION LOCATION: As marked.

PITFALLS: Fluoroscopic, CT, or EMG guidance should be used.

BTX-A DOSE: 100 U

DILUTION: 100 mU in 3 cc saline

NUMBER OF SITES: 1

FIGURE 7.18. Suggested injection site for psoas muscle.

INDICATION: Painful hip/trunk flexion.

PITFALLS: Fluoroscopic, CT, or EMG guidance should be used.

Note: Injection depth can be gauged by aiming the needle toward the top of transverse process of L4 or L5, then redirecting it laterally into the psoas muscle. Injections that are too deep may penetrate into the peritoneal cavity.

INJECTION LOCATION: Just deep to the level of the transverse spinous process of L4 or L5, as marked.

BTX-A DOSE: 100–200 U

DILUTION: 100 U in 3 cc saline

NUMBER OF SITES: 1

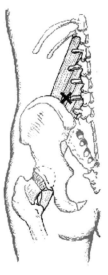

Neck

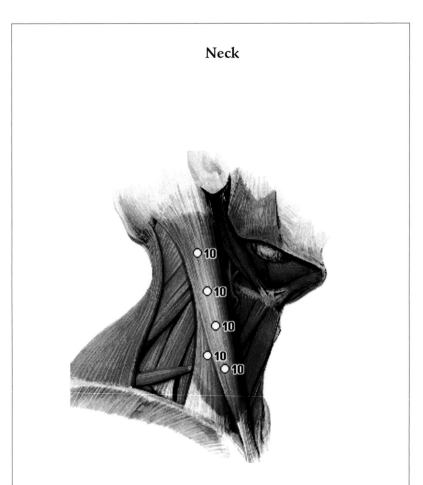

FIGURE 7.19. Suggested injection sites for the sternocleidomastoid muscle.

INDICATIONS: Painful rotation of the neck.

PITFALLS: Proximity of this muscle to vessels and pharynx.

INJECTION LOCATION: As marked, angle of the needle should be directed from medial to lateral to avoid diffusion into muscles of the larynx.

BTX-A DOSE: 50–75 U

DILUTION: 100 U in 1 cc saline

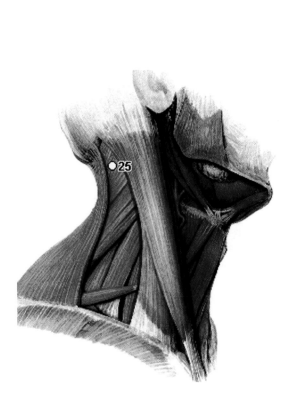

FIGURE 7.20. Suggested injection site for the splenius capitus muscle.

INDICATIONS: Painful rotation (ipsilateral) and extension of the neck

PITFALLS: Injection that is too posterior will be in trapezius; too anterior will be in sternocleidomastoid muscle.

INJECTION LOCATION: As marked.

BTX-A DOSE: 25–50 U

DILUTION: 100 U in 1 cc saline

NUMBER OF SITES: 1

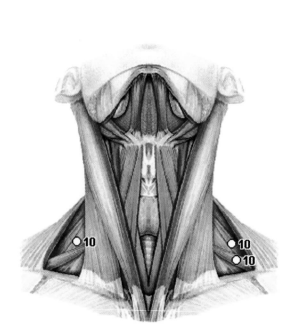

FIGURE 7.21. Suggested injection site for the scalene muscles.

INDICATION: Painful forward and lateral flexion of the neck.

PITFALLS: Proximity to vital structures (vessels and nerves); fluoroscopy and/or EMG guidance is strongly recommended.

INJECTION LOCATION: As marked. Note that for clarity, the anterior and posterior scalene injection locations are shown on the opposite side as the middle scalene injection location.

BTX-A DOSE: 30–50 U

DILUTION: 30 U in 1 cc saline

REFERENCES

Awad EA. Muscle fiber and motor endplate [letter]. *Arch Phys Med Rehabil* 61:149–190, 1980.

Awad EA, Awad OE. *Injection techniques for spasticity,* pp. 41–42. Minneapolis, MN: Author, 1993.

Borodic GE, Ferrante R, Pearce LB, Smith K. Histologic assessment of dose-related diffusion and muscle fiber response after therapeutic botulinum A toxin injections. *Mov Disord* 9:31–39, 1994.

Brans JW, de Boer IP, Aramideh M, Ongerboer de Visser BW, Speelman JD. Botulinum toxin in cervical dystonia: low dosage with electromyographic guidance *J Neurol* 242:529–523, 1995.

Brown WF, Varkey GP. The origin of spontaneous electrical activity at the end-plate zone. *Ann Neurol* 10:557–560, 1981.

Buchthal F. Spontaneous electrical activity: an overview. [Review.] *Muscle Nerve* 5:S52–S59, 1982.

Childers MK. Rationale for injection procedures for botulinum toxin type A in skeletal limb muscles. *Eur J Neurol* 4(suppl 2):37–40, 1997.

Coers C. In: *The Innervation of Muscle.* Springfield, IL: Charles C Thomas, pp. 1–20, 1959.

Halpern D. Histologic studies in animals after intramuscular neurolysis with phenol. *Arch Phys Med Rehabil* 58:438–443, 1977.

Halpern D, Meelhuysen FE. Phenol motor point block in the management of muscular hypertonia. *Arch Phys Med Rehabil* 47:659–664, 1966.

Hong CZ, Hsueh TC. Difference in pain relief after trigger point injections in myofascial pain patients with and without fibromyalgia. *Arch Phys Med Rehabil* 77:1161–1166, 1996.

Hong CZ, Simons DG. Pathophysiologic and electrophysiologic mechanisms of myofascial trigger points. [Review.] *Arch Phys Med Rehabil* 79:863–872, 1998.

Rosales RL, Arimura K, Takenaga S, Osame M. Extrafusal and intrafusal muscle effects in experimental botulinum toxin-A injection. *Muscle Nerve* 19:488–496, 1996.

Shaari CM, Sanders I. Quantifying how location and dose of botulinum toxin injections affect muscle paralysis. *Muscle Nerve* 16:964–969, 1993.

Speelman JD and Brans JW. Cervical dystonia and botulinum treatment: Is electromyographic guidance necessary? *Mov Disord* 10:802, 1995.

Wiederholt WC. "End-plate noise" in electromyography. *Neurology* 20:214–224, 1970.

CHAPTER EIGHT

Martin K. Childers

Daniel J. Wilson

DOCUMENTATION

THIS CHAPTER DESCRIBES THE INFORMATION THAT IS IMPORTANT TO DOCUMENT when evaluating and treating patients with painful conditions using botulinum toxin type A (BTX-A). This includes information such as previous treatment, response to prior treatment, medical work-up, plan for future treatment, and measures of response to treatment planned.

Measuring pain is a complex issue because of the nature of individual recognition and interpretation of pain. The complexity of evaluating pain intensity led Melzack and Wall (1965) to formulate the gate control theory of pain. This conceptual model of pain perception was expanded from a pure sensory model to a model encompassing sensory, motivational, and cognitive components. Despite an expanded understanding of the psychological basis of pain intensity, the relationship between pain and musculoskeletal pathophysiology remains in need of instruments that measure self-report and physical function.

Experts (Gracely and Dubner, 1981; Price and Harkins, 1992) have proposed criteria for ideal assessment methods that incorporate reliable, sensitive ratio scales that separately assess sensory and affective dimensions of pain. The ideal method would include data about the accuracy and reliability of patients. Some examples of self-report scales developed to estimate pain intensity using these criteria are the Verbal Rating Scale, the Visual Analog Scale, and the Numerical Rating Scale. Each of these scales was designed to measure pain intensity and provide statistical data. However, these instruments do not provide information about musculoskeletal limitations imposed by pain.

EVALUATING EFFECTS OF PAIN ON PHYSICAL FUNCTION

Assessment of range of motion using a "two inclinometer" technique is an example of a test used to evaluate the physical effects/limitations imposed by pain (Engelberg, 1988). These and other tests used to evaluate the physical effects/limitations imposed by pain are summarized in Table 8.1. While these instruments are physiologically relevant, they do not provide information about the intensity of pain perceived by the patient.

EXAMPLES OF DOCUMENTATION FOR BTX-A TREATMENT

PiqûrePerfect (Medsys Technologies; see Appendix B) is a software program that allows the clinician to document and track BTX-A injection treatments by entering information into custom templates. The documentation shown below was gathered using this program.

TABLE 8.1

Physical capacity tests used to evaluate the effects of
musculoskeletal pain and their statistical properties

Range of Motion
Two inclinometer test
  – Valid relative to lumbar flexion and extension (Mayer et al, 1985)
  – Intra- and intertester reliability established (Keeley et al, 1986)

Trunk Strength
Cybex Isokinetic Device
  – Proven validity and repeatability (Langrana and Lee, 1984; Smith et al, 1985)

Lifting Capacity
Cybex Liftask
  – Comparative norms established (Mayer et al, 1991)

PATIENT DEMOGRAPHICS

Figure 8.1 illustrates typical patient demographic data recorded at the initial clinic visit prior to treatment. The "Chart Notes" window allows the clinician to record practical information such as a reminder to get precertification numbers. Note that this program is most useful for patients who have already been identified for BTX-A treatment.

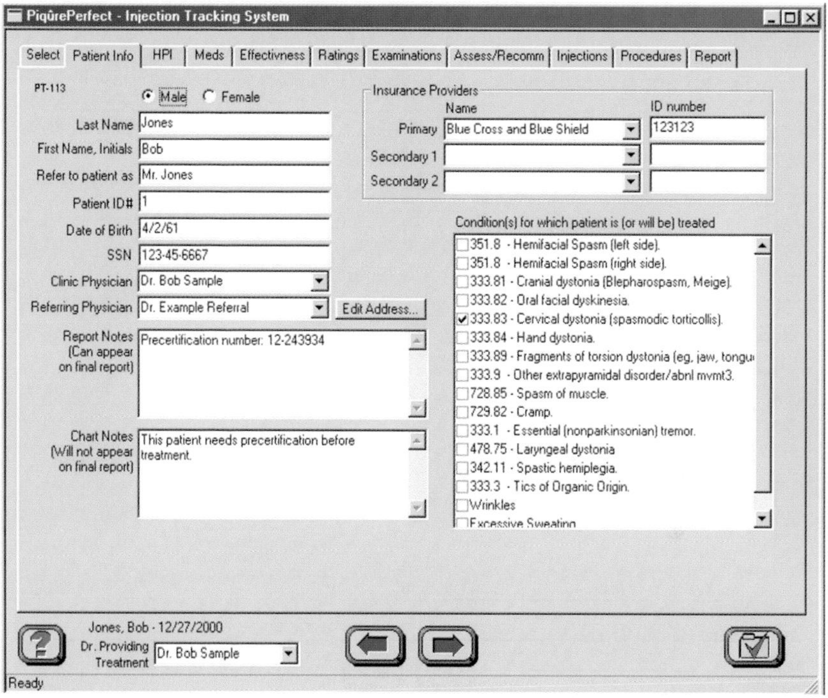

FIGURE 8.1. Typical patient intake assessment prior to treatment. Documentation using injection tracking software (PiqûrePerfect®, Medsys Technologies, Inc.).

HISTORY OF PRESENT ILLNESS

In documenting the history of present illness (Figure 8.2), it is important to note the complaint, activities that the condition interferes with, what the condition is exacerbated by, and response to previous treatment. Note that PiqûrePerfect offers stock history phrases specific to various BTX-A responsive conditions.

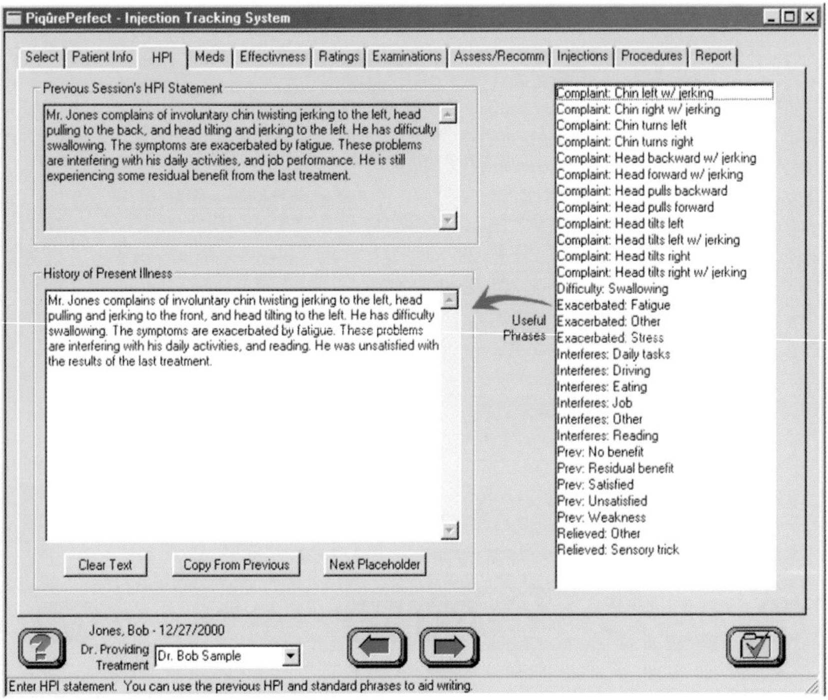

FIGURE 8.2. Typical patient history prior to treatment. Documentation using injection tracking software (PiqûrePerfect, Medsys Technologies, Inc.).

MEDICATIONS

Since evaluation of response to BTX-A treatment can be problematic, the clinician should pay careful attention to any medication changes during the treatment period. Specifically, medications such as L-DOPA that may mediate motor control, should be carefully documented (Figure 8.3).

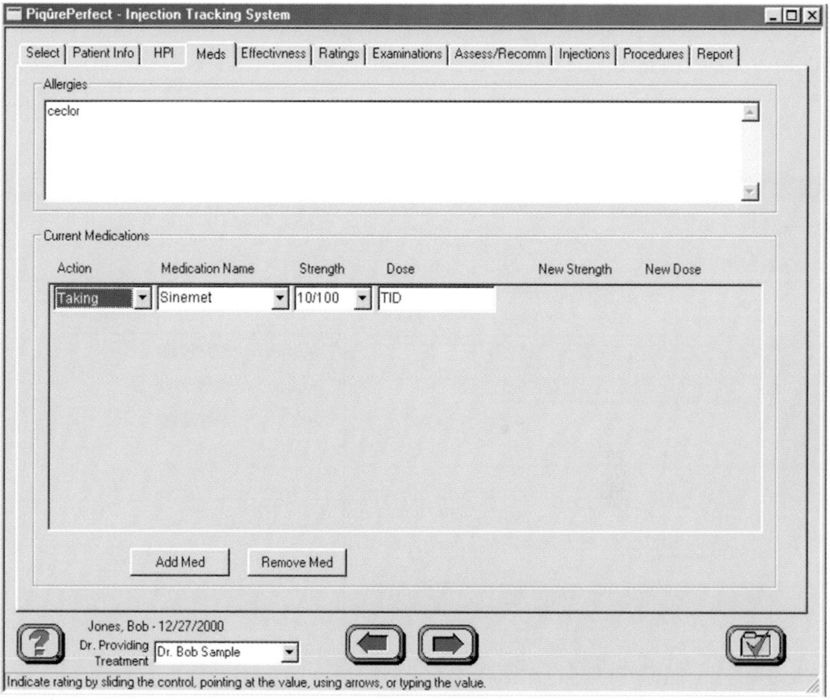

FIGURE 8.3. Medication history prior to treatment. Documentation using injection tracking software (PiqûrePerfect, Medsys Technologies, Inc.).

EFFECTIVENESS OF LAST TREATMENT

The clinical efficacy of BTX-A treatment is dose-related, not only in terms of the magnitude of response but also in the duration of action. Thus, the "Time to Benefit" and "Length of Benefit" (Figure 8.4) capture data of this dose–response relationship. For example, if a patient reports decreased clinical benefit from the previous injection session, he/she may also describe shorter duration of the treatment effects. This might indicate to the clinician that the previous dose used was too small. On the other hand, if the previous dose used was too high, unintended weakness may result. Side effects (Figure 8.4) of previous treatment should also be documented. Software such as PiqûrePerfect also allows for tracking of benefits and side effects of BTX-A therapy.

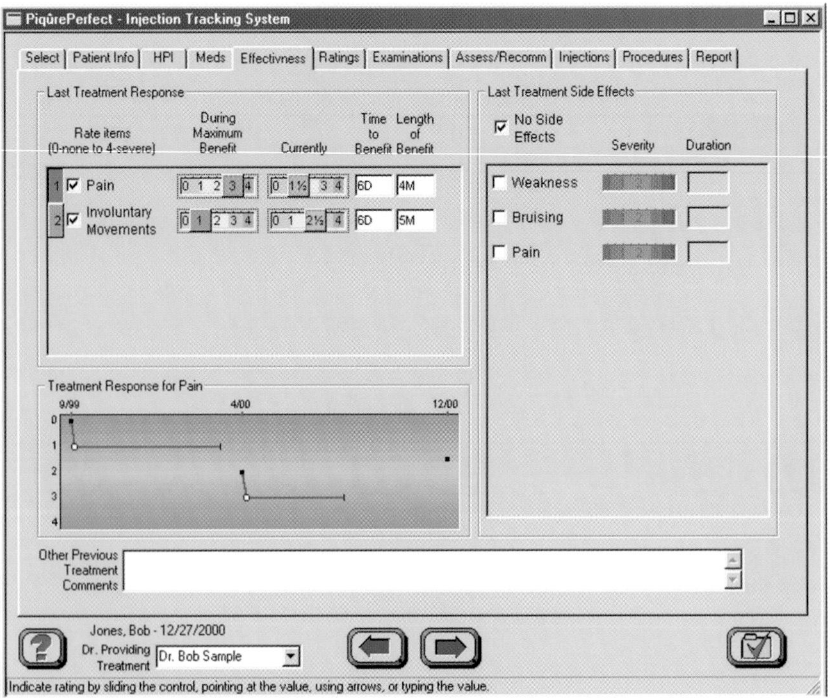

FIGURE 8.4. Clinical efficacy of BTX-A treatment. In this example, no side effects were reported. Documentation using injection tracking software (PiqûrePerfect, Medsys Technologies, Inc.).

EXAMINATION AND RATING SCALES

To determine efficacy of therapy with BTX-A, the clinician must measure and document the severity of the patient's condition under treatment. The exam should be focused on the target area(s) being considered for treatment. Because the treatment of painful conditions with BTX-A encompasses such a wide variety of circumstances, a generalized physical examination for all patients is not always sufficient. However, since many patients with disordered movement (such as cervical dystonia and spasticity) may find pain relief from BTX-A injections, standardized rating scales for a variety of BTX-A responsive conditions should be used (Figure 8.5).

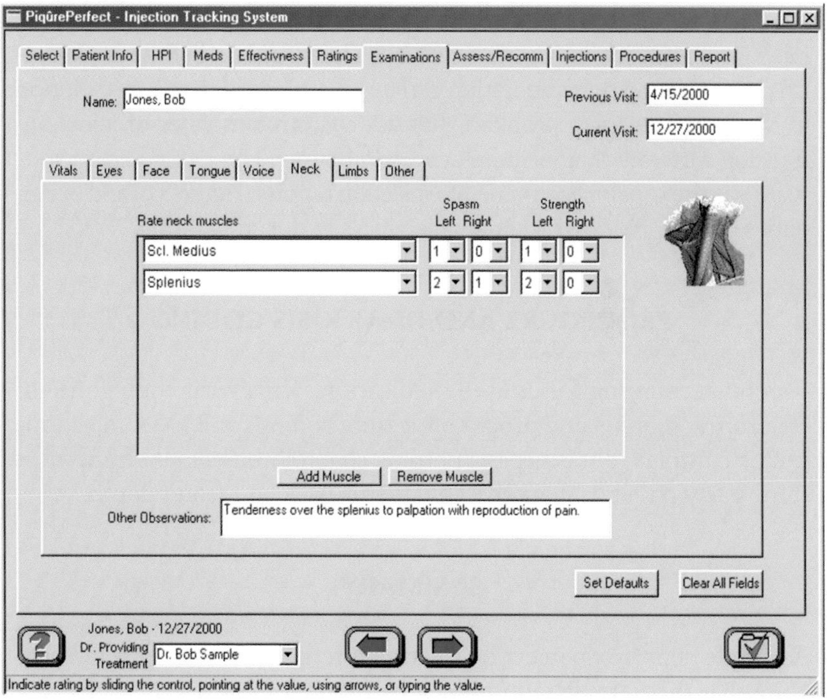

FIGURE 8.5. Examination rating. In this example, reproduction of the patient's usual pain with palpation of the splenius muscle was reported. Documentation using injection tracking software (PiqûrePerfect, Medsys Technologies, Inc.).

INFORMED CONSENT

In addition to the clinical assessment and recommendations for treatment, informed consent should be obtained in writing from the patient and documented in the medical record. It is also a good idea for family members to be informed of any material risks and given time to ask questions. The author typically waits until a subsequent clinic session before providing injections of BTX-A to allow patients and family members sufficient time to discuss and think about recommended treatment. A sample consent form is shown in Appendix C.

REPORT OF INJECTION PROCEDURES

The clinician should carefully document the medication preparation, dose, dilution, method of injection, anatomical target, and number of sites injected. Accurate records facilitated the duplication of previously successful injection sessions and may help the clinician avoid earlier methodological pitfalls. Good documentation can be an awkward task. One solution to the record-keeping problem is to use custom templates or injection-tracking software that includes anatomic figures. The PiqûrePerfect software has the capability to generate injection reports (Figure 8.6) and exemplifies one approach to accurate injection-site documentation.

PROCEDURE AND DIAGNOSIS CODING

Careful accounting for unused medication, office visit coding, use of electromyography, and proper procedure coding for BTX-A injections can be complex, but is necessary to receive reimbursement from most third-party payers. Chapter 9 covers this issue in greater depth.

SUMMARY

A sample neurotoxin injection treatment report is shown in Figure 8.6. Note that this sample report includes all the information described in this chapter including anatomical images of injection sites, dose, and target muscles. Such inclusive documentation may be helpful to referring physicians and third-party payers, and provides others with an in-depth view of the treatment approach using BTX-A.

NEUROTOXIN INJECTION TREATMENT REPORT

Patient ID:	2	Treatment Date:	12/27/2000
Patient Name:	Smith, Sarah	Previous Treatment:	5/1/2000
Date of Birth:	5/21/61	Time Between:	7.9 Months
Physician:	Dr. Bob Sample	Referred by:	Dr. Example Referral

PROCEDURES

J058—*Botulinium Toxin 40 U*
64613—*Chemodenerv, bleph/cranial, HFS (333.81,351.8)*
99213—*Office visit, established patient, level*

40 U of Botox was given (40 U injected + 0 U wasted).

HISTORY OF PRESENT ILLNESS

Ms. Smith complains of involuntary twitching on the right side of the face. The symptoms are exacerbated by fatigue, and stress. These problems are interfering with her ability to drive, and speaking. She was satisfied with the results of the last treatment. She is still experiencing some residual benefit from the last treatment.

MEDICATIONS

Allergies: *penicillin*

CURRENT MEDICATIONS

Adderall 20 mg, 1 tab prn

PREVIOUS TREATMENT*

Ms. Smith reported the onset of benefit was 4 days. During maximum benefit, she indicated that she had mild pain (rated at 1) and mild involuntary movements (rated at 0.5). The duration of benefit was reported by her as 6 months. The side effects experienced included: mild weakness (rated: 0.5) that lasted 2 days, mild bruising (rated: 0.5) that lasted 1 day and mild pain (rated: 0.5) that lasted 1 day. Currently, she is experiencing moderate pain (rated at 2.5) and moderate involuntary movements (rated at 2.5).

(continued)

FIGURE 8.6. Injection report. Documentation using injection tracking software (PiqûrePerfect, Medsys Technologies, Inc.). *Ratings are on a 4-point scale: 0 = none to 4 = severe.

RATING SCALES

Dystonia Rating Scale

MOVEMENT SCALE: Ms. Smith has mild dystonia of the eyes with frequent blinking but no prolonged spasms of eye closure. She has grimacing and other mouth movements which are present less than 50% of the time. These movements can be provoked by many different actions. Occasionally in speaking, she has slightly indistinct speech but is still easily understood. She has no dystonia of the neck, the left arm, the right arm, the trunk, the left leg or the right leg. The total score on the dystonia movement scale is 5 out of a possible 120.

DISABILITY SCALE: Her speech is somewhat indistinct but she can still be understood easily. She has no difficulty writing legibly. She can eat but is unable to use a knife. She has difficulty swallowing, and frequently chokes. She is able to take care of her personal hygienic needs independently. She can get dressed normally without assistance. She is able to walk normally. The total score on the dystonia disability scale is 5 out of a possible 30.

EXAMINATION

Face: There was increased blinking in the right eye. There was no decreased blinking. There was no increased blinking with squeezing of the lids in either eye. Apraxia of the lid opening was present in the right eye. There was no synkinesis of lid blinking and lateral movements of the ipsilateral side of the mouth on either side of the face. Flurries of twitches of the eyelids accompanied by a pulling of the corner of the mouth laterally were not present.

ASSESSMENT

Diagnosis: 351.8—*Hemifacial spasm (right side).*
Ms. Smith is appropriate for reinjection of neurotoxin.

RECOMMENDATIONS

Ms. Smith signed the consent form. The risks and nature of the procedure were explained and she agreed to have the procedure performed. Ms. Smith is to return when benefit has diminished.

INJECTION SUMMARY

Ms. Smith received 40 U of Botox in 8 injections. The following muscles were injected:

Amount	Muscle
5 U	*Epicranius - Occipitofrontalis Venter Frontalis (right)*
15 U	*Orbicularis Oculi (right)*
5 U	*Levator Labii Superioris (right)*
5 U	*Zygomaticus Minor (right)*
5 U	*Masseter (right)*
5 U	*Risorius (right)*

The specific injection sites and amounts are as shown in the following diagram(s):

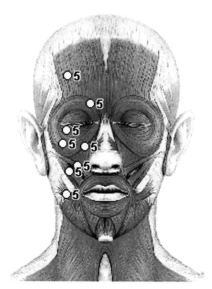

All examinations, ratings, assessments, recommendations and procedures were done by Dr. Bob Sample.

Signed: _____ Date: _____

REFERENCES

Engelberg A. American Medical Association guides to the evaluation of permanent impairment. Chicago: American Medical Association, 1988.

Gracely RH, Dubner R. Pain assessment in humans: A reply to Hall. *Pain* 11:109–120, 1981.

Keeley J, Mayer TG, Cox R, Gatchel RJ, Smith J, Mooney V. Quantification of lumbar function. Part 5: Reliability of range-of-motion measures in the sagittal plane and an in vivo torso rotation measurement technique. *Spine* 11:31–35, 1986.

Langrana NA, Lee CK. Isokinetic evaluation of trunk muscles. *Spine* 9:171–175, 1984.

Mayer T, Gatchel R, Keeley J, Mayer H, Richland D. Building industrial databases: Physical capacity measurements specific to major job categories in U.S. railroads. *Proc Int Soc* 1991.

Mayer T, Kishino N, Keeley J, Mayer H, Mooney V. Using physical measures to assess low back pain. *J Musculoskel Med* 6:44–59, 1985.

Medsys Technologies, Inc. PiqûrePerfect®. St Louis, MO. www.medsystechnologies.com

Melzack R, Wall PD. Pain mechanisms: A new theory. *Science* 150:971–979, 1965.

Price DD, Harkins SW. Psychophysical approaches to pain measurement and assessment. In: Turk DC, Melzak R (eds.). *Handbook of Pain Assessment.* New York: Guilford Press, pp. 111–134, 1992.

Smith SS, Mayer TG, Gatchel RJ, Becker TJ. Quantification of lumbar function. Part 1: Isometric and multispeed isokinetic trunk strength measures in sagittal and axial planes in normal subjects. *Spine* 10:757–764, 1985.

CHAPTER NINE

Diane Simison

OBTAINING REIMBURSEMENT

THIS CHAPTER DISCUSSES COVERAGE AND REIMBURSEMENT BY THIRD-PARTY payers for botulinum toxin type A (BTX-A; Botox, Allergan, Inc.). Botox is the only botulinum toxin type A approved by the FDA at this time. While the FDA has approved a botulinum toxin type B formulation, the approved indication is limited specifically to cervical dystonia. As other botulinum toxins enter the market, each may have slightly different coverage policies and reimbursement mechanisms based on specific approved labeling, clinical characteristics, and formulations. Most major third-party payers will provide coverage and reimbursement for botulinum toxin type A. However, obtaining reimbursement will require your attention for the following reasons:

- The rules and requirements for obtaining coverage and reimbursement vary by payer.
- Reimbursement amounts are different for each payer.
- Reimbursement rules and amounts can vary for each setting of care (eg, physician's office, hospital outpatient clinic, ambulatory surgical center).

The following pages contain a general overview of payer policies on coverage and reimbursement for BTX-A treatment, important considerations in preparing claims, and additional information specific to coverage and reimbursement in various treatment setttings

To obtain reimbursement from a third-part payer, your patient must have an insurance benefit that will include coverage for BTX-A treatment. You should verify the patient's benefits and obtain instructions from the payer for filing the reimbursement claim. Precise instructions can be obtained from the patient's insurance company.

A REVIEW OF THIRD-PARTY PAYER REQUIREMENTS

In this section, the important aspects of obtaining coverage and reimbursement for BTX-A treatment from third-party payers are reviewed. Since Medicare has the most specific requirements, the discussion for this payer is more detailed.

Medicare: Insurer of Those Over Age 65 and the Disabled

Since BTX-A treatment will be administered in the outpatient setting, it will fall under Part B of the Medicare benefit. About 25 different Medicare carriers administer the Medicare outpatient benefit and process claims for 56 states or state regions. A separate policy or guideline has been issued by Medicare carriers for coverage and reimbursement for BTX-A treatment for each state or state region.

- BTX-A treatment will be reimbursed when administered by a physician to a Medicare-eligible patient.
- Regional Medicare carriers have some latitude in determining coverage policies; therefore there is some variability in the coverage for BTX-A treatment for pain diagnoses under Medicare.
- Reimbursement will be triggered by the presence of approved CPT procedure codes and ICD-9 diagnosis codes on the CMS 1500 claim form; Medicare does not provide prior authorization of services.
- BTX-A treatment will be reimbursed when administered in various outpatient settings (including the physician's office, hospital outpatient clinics, ambulatory surgery centers, and

pain clinics), but not for all diagnoses and procedures.

- BTX-A should be billed using code J0585 (botulinum toxin type A, per unit).
- Medicare reimbursement for BTX-A treatment will be 80% of the allowable amount; the patient pays the other 20%.
- The Medicare allowable amount for BTX-A treatment currently is 95% of the average wholesale price (AWP) per vial of drug.

Diagnosis and Procedure Codes Are Important to Reimbursement

Medicare will reimburse the cost of BTX-A treatment when it is used with a covered ("payable") diagnosis. Covered diagnoses will be listed in the local coverage policies issued by the Medicare carriers. If BTX-A treatment is medically necessary for a diagnosis not listed as covered, you should submit documentation supporting the medical necessity and clinical literature supporting the use to the carrier (Bickerton et al, 1997; Childers, 1997, 1998; Shaari and Sanders, 1993).

As with ICD-9 diagnosis codes, Medicare policies list the CPT procedure codes for which BTX-A treatment will be reimbursed. Medicare does not currently list CPT code 20550 as covered in policies for BTX-A treatment.

A list of codes that might be used for pain indications is shown in Table 9.1.

Coverage Guidelines—ICD-9 and CPT Code Pairings

In many cases, Medicare provides guidelines for coverage of BTX-A treatment. For Medicare, a coverage guideline consists of a CPT code that is payable when used with specified ICD-9 diagnoses. If a Medicare carrier has implemented coverage guidelines, the paired codes are listed in the Medicare policy.

Electromyography Procedure Coding

Medicare will pay for electromyography when used in association with a BTX-A injection. Medicare policies list covered electromyography codes. Those most frequently covered appear in Table 9.1.

TABLE 9.1

*Pain-related CPT and ICD-9 codes approved by most
Medicare Part B carriers*

ICD-9 Diagnosis Codes

728.8	Other disorders of muscle, ligament, fascia, spasm of muscle
333-333.9	Dystonias
342-342.1	Hemiplegia and hemiparesis
343-343.9	Cerebral palsy

CPT Procedure Codes

64640	Destruction by neurolytic agent; other peripheral nerve or branch
64612	Destruction by neurolytic agent; muscles enervated by facial nerve
64613	Destruction by neurolytic agent; cervical spinal muscles
64614	Chemodenervation of the muscle(s); extremity(s), and/or trunk muscle(s)
95861	Needle electromyography; two extremities

Coding Guideline

728.85 with 64640

Electromyography

95860	Needle electromyography, one extremity
95867	Needle electromyography, cranial nerve supplied muscles, unilateral
95868	Needle electromyography, cranial nerve supplied muscles, bilateral
95869	Needle electromyography, limited study of specific muscles (to be replaced with code 95870)
95870	Needle electromyography, other than paraspinal muscles

Proper Use of Modifiers Is Essential to Medicare Reimbursement

Modifiers document specific information regarding the procedure, such as the anatomic area of the body being treated (anatomical) or aspects of the procedure itself that have been altered (procedural). Modifiers are to be recorded on the claim form.

In the case of Medicare, correct use of modifiers can be associated with higher reimbursement rates, and incorrect use can be associated with claims denial or "downcoding" (where a lesser amount of reimbursement is paid).

Medicare Policies Contain Instructions on Dosage and Number of Injections

Medicare policies may set reimbursement limits on the amount of a drug to be used for types of muscles or on the number of injections per site. Medicare defines a "site" as noncontiguous muscle groups. Only one injection will be reimbursed per site.

The dosage limits may specify the amount of the drug that is reimbursable for muscles of various sizes, or the number of injections that may be reimbursable over a certain period of time.

You should obtain the payer's written policy regarding limitations on dosage or number of injections of botulinum toxin, and follow the coding instructions accordingly.

Medicare Will Pay for Discarded BTX-A Under Certain Conditions

Medicare carriers will pay for BTX-A that must be discarded, and has established certain rules for how the wastage is to be recorded. You should obtain a copy of the payer's instructions that describe how the discarded amount is to be billed and documented in the patient's medical record.

Medicare Requires Documentation

Medicare requires that the medical necessity for a procedure be documented in the patient's record. Occasionally, a payer will require the submission of a letter of medical necessity prior to approval of payment.

In these cases, you should submit a letter of medical necessity for treatment with BTX-A to the insurance plan medical director. Your letter should include the following information:

- Reason for treatment
- Physical examination findings
- Impression—including primary and secondary diagnosis and their effects
- Prior treatments
- Plan and recommendations—including why BTX-A treatment is being prescribed, and injection areas
- Conclusion—including diagnosis codes, dosage, areas of injection, and follow-up needed

MEDICAID

Medicaid is a joint federal and state entitlement program providing health care benefits for low-income individuals who are aged, disabled, or blind. The coverage amount of reimbursement, as well as how BTX-A treatment must be obtained, will vary among the states.

- Regardless of the treatment setting, BTX-A treatment will usually be covered under the Physician Services Program; in some cases, it may be covered under the Outpatient Prescription Drug Program.
- Physicians will be reimbursed for BTX-A based on the average wholesale price (AWP) minus a percentage (usually about 10%); reimbursement for other procedures is provided in a variety of ways, such as by fee schedule, actual cost, or an approved charge.
- Prior approval of BTX-A treatment may be necessary.

In some states, BTX-A must be billed and paid under the patient's Medicaid outpatient pharmacy drug benefit. You must check with your state Medicaid office to determine if this is required in your state. If it is required, the patient must pick up BTX-A at a Medicaid-approved pharmacy and bring it to the physician's office for injection. The pharmacy will bill Medicaid for the BTX-A.

COMMERCIAL AND MANAGED CARE INSURERS

Commercial and managed care payers will cover BTX-A treatment for FDA-approved uses and for some other uses as well when medically necessary and when the use is supported in the clinical literature.

Many commercial insurers have adopted the principles of managed care, where the patient must see a physician in the payer network and treatment may be restricted by a treatment guideline. In all cases, the insurance plan requirements must be determined prior to treatment with botulinum toxin.

- Coverage and reimbursement will vary based on the provisions of the patient's insurance plan and the setting in which BTX-A is administered.
- Prior authorization, or precertification, of the use of BTX-A will be necessary in many cases.
- Documentation of medical necessity will be required for prior authorization.
- Coverage for BTX-A treatment may depend on the plan formulary.
- The insurer's medical director often determines coverage for expensive pharmaceuticals, after reviewing other treatment options and the medical necessity.

If a treatment is given before required precertification is obtained, the payer may deny coverage and the patient may be required to pay the cost of botulinum toxin. Therefore, it should be determined before treatment if prior authorization is required. A call may be made to the patient's insurance plan to obtain this information.

WORKERS' COMPENSATION

Each state has a program to pay for treatment of workers injured during job performance. The requirements and characteristics of each state program are different, but there are some similarities.

- Return to work is the goal for all workers' compensation programs.

- All necessary health care is paid for if it is medically necessary.
- Some states will require precertification for treatments with BTX-A.
- Most states reimburse for medical services based on fee schedules.
- Some states have treatment guidelines in which therapy must be listed prior to coverage.

Some workers' compensation programs have established treatment guidelines and have referenced treatment with botulinum toxin. For example, BTX-A is referenced in the lower extremity treatment guideline adopted by workers' compensation in Texas. You can obtain this information from each state's workers' compensation agency.

COVERAGE AND BILLING FOR BTX-A TREATMENT— MECHANISMS OF PAYMENT

The requirements and process for obtaining payment for BTX-A treatment will vary among payers and according to the setting of care in which treatment is delivered.

Payers recognize whether a claim is payable and enforce payment restrictions through a review of the claim. Those components of the claim that are important in obtaining payment for BTX-A treatment are reviewed below.

IMPORTANT ISSUES FOR USE OF BTX-A TO TREAT PAIN

Trigger Point Injections

You should determine whether you are treating the trigger point or whether you are treating the surrounding spasm. You must examine your coding options prior to selecting a code that best represents the nature of the treatment.

To date, no Medicare carrier policy lists CPT codes 20550 (injection, tendon sheath, ligament, trigger point) or diagnosis 729.1 as covered codes for BTX-A injections.

Special Payer Rules for the Pain Clinic

Reimbursement of the Ambulatory Surgery Center by Medicare

If you are administering treatment with BTX-A in a pain clinic rather than in your office, the clinic must be classified as a place of service on the HCFA 1500 claim form. This code provides the appropriate coverage and reimbursement information for the services rendered.

Most pain clinics will be classified as an ambulatory surgery center (ASC), a hospital outpatient department, or an outpatient rehabilitation clinic. Only you can determine which classification is correct. The facility and the physician will both receive payments for treatment in these settings.

Ambulatory surgery centers are paid prospectively. If the treatment is one approved by Medicare to be given in an ambulatory surgery center, the CPT procedure is grouped into one of eight ASC payment groups. The group assignment determines the amount that Medicare pays for facility services furnished in connection with a covered procedure. Currently, none of the CPT procedures used for the injections of BTX-A are included in the list of approved procedures. Thus, no payment will be made to the ASC if BTX-A is injected in an ASC. However, the physician services are reimbursable by Medicare, as is the charge for the BTX-A, if it is included in the physicians's bill.

If the CPT procedure is grouped into an ASC payment but delivered in a hospital outpatient department instead of an ambulatory surgery center, the facility payment is the lesser of a blended rate (42% of the hospital's reasonable costs or charges and 58% of the ASC payment rate). Pharmaceuticals used in ASC-approved procedures performed in the hospital outpatient department are generally covered separately, and charges for them are used in the calculation of the payment rate.

HOW TO OBTAIN INFORMATION ABOUT COVERAGE AND PAYMENT FOR BTX-A TREATMENT

Following are sources for information about coverage and reimbursement for BTX-A used to treat pain:

YOUR MEDICARE PART B CARRIER
You can obtain the policy detailing requirements for obtaining

reimbursement for BTX-A treatment from your Medicare Part B carrier. If you do not have the name and address of the carrier, you can locate it on the HCFA website at http://www.hcfa.gov.

YOUR PATIENT'S INSURANCE COMPANY

The patient's insurance company will verify the patient's benefit so that you can be sure that reimbursement will be forthcoming. The insurance company will also be able to tell you if precertification is required, if there are other requirements for submitting claims, and what the reimbursement amount will be.

REFERENCES

Bickerton LE, Agur AM, Ashby P. Flexor digitorum superficialis: Locations of individual muscle bellies for botulinum toxin injections. *Muscle Nerve* 20:1041–1043, 1997.

Childers MK. Rationale for injection procedures for botulinum toxin type A in skeletal limb muscles. *Eur J Neurol* 4(Suppl 2):37–40, 1997.

Childers MK, Kornegay JN, Aoki R, Otaviani L, Bogan DJ, Petroski G. Evaluating motor end-plate-targeted injections of botulinum toxin type A in a canine model. *Muscle Nerve* 21:653–655, 1998.

Shaari CM andSanders I. Quantifying how location and dose of botulinum toxin injections affect muscle paralysis. *Muscle Nerve* 16:964–969, 1993.

NEUROMUSCULAR PHYSIOLOGY FOR BOTULINUM TOXIN TYPE A USERS

KEY FACTS

- Acetylcholine has broad functions as a neurotransmitter throughout the peripheral nervous system.
- Botulinum toxin type A blocks the release of acetylcholine.
- Physicians can exploit the unique physiological actions of acetylcholine blockade using botulinum toxin type A.
- Understanding how and where acetylcholine functions in the body is key.

ACETYLCHOLINE IN MUSCULAR CONTRACTION

Acetylcholine (ACh) (Figure A.1) is the major neurotransmitter involved in skeletal muscle contraction. The action of acetylcholine in skeletal muscle occurs at the neuromuscular junction. ACh enters the synapse at this junction through its calcium-activated release from the presynaptic membrane. It then binds to nicotinic receptors on the postsynaptic muscle membrane. These nicotinic receptors, a type of ionotropic receptor, allow transport of sodium and potassium ions across the

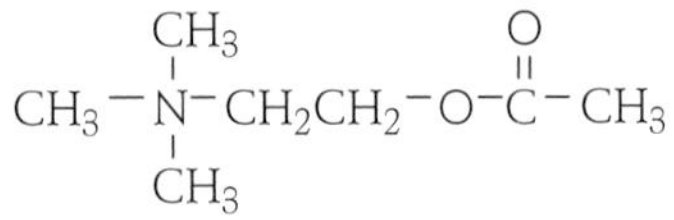

$$CH_3 - \overset{\displaystyle \overset{CH_3}{|}}{\underset{\displaystyle \underset{CH_3}{|}}{N}} - CH_2CH_2 - O - \overset{\displaystyle \overset{O}{\|}}{C} - CH_3$$

FIGURE A.1. Chemical structure of ACh.

postsynaptic cell membrane when activated by ACh. The entry of sodium causes depolarization of the cell membrane and generation of an end-plate potential. The end-plate potential initiates propagation of an action potential along the cell membrane of the skeletal muscle cell and ultimately skeletal muscle contraction.

Botulinum toxin type A (BTX-A) prevents presynaptic ACh release by modulating a membrane-bound protein, SNAP 25, which results in the inhibition of the calcium-activated release of ACh. Other serotypes of the botulinum toxins (serotypes are designated A–F) act on different neuronal proteins, such as syntaxin or vesicle-associated membrane protein.

ACh Relaxes Smooth Muscle in Some Tissues

In some types of smooth muscle that line the interior of blood vessels (arterioles of some tissue), acetylcholine may cause smooth muscle relaxation. When ACh binds to muscarinic receptors found on blood vessel endothelial cells, the resulting increase in intracellular calcium produces relaxation. (Note that calcium is increased in the endothelial cells, not the smooth muscle cells.) Muscarinic receptors are considered metabatropic, since they act by metabolic pathways involving phospholipases. Calcium acts as a second messenger, triggering the release of a nitric oxide that diffuses out of the endothelial cell and into the smooth muscle surrounding the blood vessels. The effect of nitric oxide is to relax smooth muscle.

ACh Contracts Smooth Muscle in Other Tissues

Paradoxically, when ACh binds onto other kinds of smooth muscle cell receptors, such as found in the gastrointestinal tract or around the urinary bladder detrussor, muscle contraction results. When ACh binds to muscarinic receptors in these smooth muscle cells, it increases intracellular calcium and produces contraction. Calcium acts together with calmodulin to add a high-energy phosphate bond onto myosin, a muscle protein. Phosphorylation of myosin triggers an interaction of myosin with actin resulting in muscle contraction.

ACh Has Other Functions in the Peripheral Nervous System

Similar to ACh's action at the skeletal muscle nicotinic receptor, the action of ACh binding onto nicotinic receptors in preganglionic sympathetic synapses results in the opening of membrane pores. Opening pores in the preganglionic synapse of the sympathetic system also allows passage of sodium and potassium ions through the cell membrane. Passage of sodium, in particular, depolarizes the postsynaptic nerve cell, and generates an action potential.

HOW BTX-A MIGHT BE USED AT PREGANGLIONIC SYMPATHETIC SYNAPSES

Reflex sympathetic dystrophy of the upper limb is one such example of a condition that might respond to blocking ACh at the preganglionic sympathetic synapse. If the portion of the stellate ganglion (Figure A.2) of the sympathetic chain that innervates the upper limb could be safely localized, and the clinical response with the injection of a short-acting anticholinergic agent (like atracurium) was tested, injection of a very small amount of BTX-A might prove beneficial. The advantage to such treatment would be a longer duration of action than "stellate ganglion blocks" done with sodium channel blockers and steroids. The potential risks would be those associated with blocking any tonic actions of the cervical sympathetic ganglia on viscera that it innervates. However, since the predominate tonic autonomic influence on the heart is parasympathetic, it seems unlikely that removal of any tonic sympathetic influence would be undesirable. Research in animal models might further elucidate any potential side effects of BTX-A in such a setting prior to a clinical trial. Alternatively (see Chapter 2), a subcutaneous injection of BTX-A could target the nociceptive nerves in the skin and downregulate the amount of pain signal.

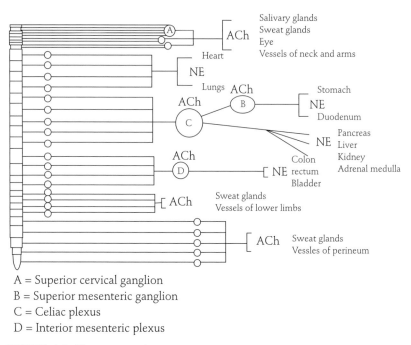

A = Superior cervical ganglion
B = Superior mesenteric ganglion
C = Celiac plexus
D = Interior mesenteric plexus

FIGURE A.2. The autonomic nervous system.

Role of ACh in Preganglionic Parasympathetic Nerve Transmission

Similar to its action in the sympathetic system, ACh is the major neurotransmitter involved in preganglionic parasympathetic synapses. ACh acts on nicotinic (ionotropic) receptors to open membrane pores, thereby allowing passage of sodium and potassium ions. It is the passage of these ions that recapitulates the action potential originating in the preganglionic nerve.

Uses of BTX-A at Preganglionic Parasympathetic Synapses

Clinicians might also exploit properties of BTX-A at preganglionic parasympathetic synapses. In fact, one such clinical report (Sherman et al, 1995), investigated injection of BTX-A into the celiac plexus (Figure A.2), a parasympathetic preganglionic region that innervates much of the gastrointestinal tract, including the pancreas. The hypothesis was that inhibition of autonomic stimulation would decrease the pain of chronic pancreatitis. While the results of this small study were mixed, the rationale for application of agents that block the action of ACh in this setting appears to be reasonable. Other painful conditions associated with overactivity of the parasympathetic nervous system might be amenable to local treatment with BTX-A. Further clinical research is needed in this area to fully explore these possibilities.

Role of ACh in Postganglionic Parasympathetic Nerve Transmission

Again, ACh is the major neurotransmitter involved in parasympathetic nerve transmission at the postganglionic synapse. Recall that in the parasympathetic system, the postganglionic nerve is relatively short, compared with the longer preganglionic nerve. In smooth muscle tissue innervated by parasympathetic nerve endings, ACh acts on muscarinic (metabatropic) receptors to increase the concentration of intracellular calcium activating the contractile system of smooth muscle.

How BTX-A Might Be Used at Postganglionic Parasympathetic Synapses

Clinicians can exploit the physiology of ACh at the postganglionic parasympathetic synapses by blocking ACh release at the target origin. One such example is seen in a condition of excessive secretion by the sweat glands, known as hyperhidrosis. For some unfortunate individuals, this excessive sweating about the axilla or palms can result in embarrassing or disabling conditions. Subcutaneous injection of 25–50 mU of BTX-A into the axillary area can alleviate hyperhidrosis for weeks or months (see Chapter 1).

In some patients, such as children with cerebral palsy, excessive salivation is a considerable problem for caretakers. Excessive salivation is caused by dysregulation of parasympathetic outflow to the salivary glands, which normally produce their own weight in saliva each minute. Since the rate of saliva production is proportional to the blood flow to the glands (regulated by the parasympathetic system), decreasing blood flow should decrease saliva production. Yet, systemic treatment with anticholinergic medications often results in drowsiness, constipation, and other undesirable side effects.

However, BTX-A may offer positive response without negative, systemic side effects. Submandibular injections of 5–10 mU BTX-A for involuntary oral-lingual movements may result in diminished outflow of saliva. This is a desirable side effect in many instances, since these individuals also have excessive salivation. Further research would be helpful to more fully investigate the effectiveness of BTX-A treatment for conditions of excessive saliva secretions.

BOTULINUM TOXIN DOES NOT BLOCK ACTION POTENTIALS IN SENSORY NERVES

The primary ions (sodium and potassium) involved in transmission of an action potential in a sensory nerve do not involve ACh. Thus, BTX-A does not affect sensory nerve action potentials. Clinicians may take advantage of this property of BTX-A. For example, in painful foot conditions associated with "alpha rigidity," a type of involuntary muscle contraction of muscles of the calf (sometimes called dystonia or spasticity), physicians may inject the tibial nerve with phenol in order to decrease the nerve supply to the offending muscles. A disadvantage to "phenol neurolysis" is that phenol affects both the sensory and motor nerves. The patient may risk losing sensation to the area supplied by the sensory nerve, or even develop painful dysesthesias in the area supplied by the sensory nerve. BTX-A offers the advantage of being selective for ACh alone, thus sparing any sensory nerve involvement. However, BTX-A might affect special nociceptive neurons that signal painful sensations. See Chapter 2 for details for more information about this mechanism.

BTX-A MAY BE MORE EFFECTIVE IN SLOW TWITCH COMPARED WITH FAST TWITCH MUSCLE

Recall that slow twitch (type I) muscle differs fundamentally from fast twitch (type II) muscle in both structure and function. Type I muscle derives energy from adenosine triphosphate (ATP) in a molecular pathway that uses oxygen as an important source of electrons. These electrons are used to create high-energy chemical bonds between phosphate and adenosine. This process of oxidative phosphorylation (adding phosphate to adenosine to create ATP) involves myoglobin, an oxygen carrier in muscle cells that imparts a dark red color to type I muscle. Alternatively, type II muscle derives energy from ATP using glycolysis, a pathway that does not require oxygen (or myoglobin). Thus, type II muscle is lighter in color than type I muscle.

BTX-A seems to be more effective in weakening slow twitch, type I, muscle fibers when compared with type II muscle fibers. This observation might be clinically useful when injecting BTX-A into muscles of the leg, such as the gastroc-soleus complex. Not only is the soleus muscle primarily composed of type I muscle fibers but, as a food animal researcher observed, muscle lying "closer to the bone" appears to have a greater number of type I fibers when compared with muscle not so "close to the bone." This may be due to the way muscle fibers are used in posture and support. This observation has led the author to target injections of BTX-A into regions of postural muscles that lie closer to the bone whenever possible. Further research in animal models may clarify the clinical usefulness of this curious observation.

In summary, ACh has broad functions as a neurotransmitter throughout the body. Understanding how and where ACh functions in both the autonomic nervous system and in skeletal muscle is important to clinicians who wish to exploit the unique action of BTX-A on ACh blockade. While the pharmacologic action of BTX-A is specific, the broad function of ACh in autonomic ganglia and nicotinic receptors in skeletal muscle allows for an array of clinical applications.

Clinical examples of how BTX-A could be used may be seen in reflex sympathetic dystrophy, chronic pancreatitis, hyperhidrosis, excessive salivation, dystonia, and spasticity. Additionally, targeting injections of BTX-A toward postural muscles lying "closer to the bone" might be beneficial.

ADDITIONAL SOURCES OF INFORMATION

INJECTION TRACKING AND DOCUMENTATION SOFTWARE
PiqûrePerfect
Medsys Technologies, Inc.
7777 Bonhomme Ave. Suite 1700
St Louis, MO 63105 USA
314-725-4626 or 866-725-2828
http://www.medsystechnologies.com

PORTABLE AUDIO EMG UNITS
Portable audio EMG
Allergan BOTOX® EMG Amplifier
Allergan Customer Service Department
1-800-377-7790
Price: Approx. $750 (US)

PORTABLE NERVE STIMULATORS/TENS
Nerve stimulators and pain management instruments:
Life Tech, Inc.
http://www.life-tech.com

2 CHANNEL TENS UNIT:
Intelect® TENS unit $79.00
Rallis Corp.
1-800-852-8898
http://www.rallis.com

VIDEO AND MONOGRAPH INFORMATION

Emerging Treatment Options for Myofascial Pain Syndromes (video)
DISCOVERY INTERNATIONAL
520 Lake Cook Road, Suite 250
Deerfield, IL 60015 USA
1-847-374-4600
1-847-374-4650 (fax)
http://www.discovery-intl.com

INJECTION TRAINING WORKSHOPS/SEMINARS

SOCIETY FOR PAIN PRACTICE MANAGEMENT
http://www.sppm.org

DANNEMILLER MEMORIAL EDUCATIONAL FOUNDATION
12500 Network Boulevard, Suite 101
San Antonio, TX 78249-3302 USA
1-800-328-2308
1-210-641-8329 (fax)
http://www.pain.com

WE MOVE—WORLDWIDE EDUCATION AND AWARENESS FOR
MOVEMENT DISORDERS
Mount Sinai Medical Center
One Gustave L. Levy Place Box 1052
New York, NY 10029 USA
1-800-437-MOV2
1-212-987-7363 (fax)
http://www.wemove.org

AMERICAN ACADEMY OF PHYSICAL MEDICINE AND REHABILITATION
(AAPM&R)
One IBM Plaza, Suite 2500
Chicago, IL 60611-3604 USA
1-312-464-9700
1-312-464-0227 (fax)
http://www.aapmr.org

THE EDITOR MAY BE CONTACTED AT THE FOLLOWING ADDRESS:
Martin K. Childers, D.O.
Associate Professor
Department of Physical Medicine and Rehabilitation
University of Missouri-Columbia
Columbia, MO 65212 USA
Email: childersmk@health.missouri.edu

SAMPLE CONSENT FORM

BOTULINUM TOXIN TYPE A INJECTION FOR TREATMENT OF DYSTONIA, SPASTICITY, OR PAINFUL SYNDROMES

Dystonia is a neurologic disorder manifested by involuntary, sustained contractions (spasms) of muscles producing abnormal postures. Injections of botulinum toxin type A (Botox®), a protein that causes temporary weakness of the injected muscles, may provide effective relief for dystonia, hemifacial spasm (involuntary twitching of one side of the face), spasticity and other painful conditions due to involuntary muscle contractions. Studies involving many patients have demonstrated the safety and effectiveness of this form of treatment.

Botulinum toxin type A has been approved by the FDA for treatment of blepharospasm and hemifacial spasm, cervical dystonia, and pain related to cervical dystonia but not for spasticity or other muscle pain. However, the American Academy of Neurology has deemed this drug safe and effective in the treatment of oromandibular, cervical, spasmodic, and focal dystonia. In addition, the National Institutes of

continued

Health has also issued a consensus statement that this drug is effective and safe in treating these disorders.

In addition to dystonia, recent clinical reports in the medical literature indicate that botulinum toxin type A treatments are safe and effective in the treatment of muscle spasticity (involuntary spasms often seen after spinal cord injury, head injury, and other neurologic disorders). Patients that have had head injuries and strokes often have symptoms with elements of both spasticity and dystonia.

Alternatives to botulinum toxin type A therapy include medications taken by mouth such as diazepam, benztropine, clonazepam, baclofen, and others. Additionally, certain physical therapies may be beneficial in the disorder as well.

You may be videotaped prior to and while receiving the medication. By signing this consent form, you give your permission to have Dr. _____ or his/her assistants, make photographs, videotapes, and/or recordings of these injections, under the condition that these photographs, etc., will be used in the interest of medical teaching, research, or health science. These photographs, tapes or recordings and information relating to your case may be published and republished in professional journals or medical books.

The procedure will consist of the following: You will receive the botulinum toxin type A by injection into the muscle through the skin. The skin will be cleaned with an alcohol pad, and the site to be injected may be determined by using a small electric stimulator that is connected to a battery or a larger machine that is called an EMG machine. This allows the physician to correctly localize the proper area of the muscle to inject. A small electric current may applied onto the surface of the skin or just beneath the surface of the skin with a small, sterilized needle. You will usually receive three needle sticks to each muscle for even distribution of the drug, and approximately 0.3 cc of fluid (less than a teaspoon) will be injected with each needle insertion.

Botulinum toxin type A may relieve symptoms for three to six months. You may notice some improvement within the next 72 hours but may not notice anything for up to two weeks. If at any time you are uncomfortable during the procedure, please let us know.

Potential benefits of this treatment would include reduction in painful spasms, increased ability to range a joint such as the ankle, knee, or arm, potential to increase the speed of walking and other functional abilities, and potential for certain physical therapies to be performed more easily, such as splinting and casting.

There are risks involved in botulinum toxin type A injections. Common side effects include muscle weakness that may affect function of the limb treated, local bruising, and discomfort at the injection site. There are other conditions listed below in which these injections are performed. The *common side effects* related to the following disorders and their treatment include:

For treatment of Blepharospasm (involuntary eye closing):
- ptosis (eyelid drooping)
- diplopia (double vision)
- burning and pain
- eyelid swelling and bruising
- tearing

For treatment of Oromandibular dystonia:
- dysphasia (swallowing and chewing difficulties)
- dysarthria (talking difficulty)
- hoarseness
- drooling

For treatment of Cervical dystonia:
- dysphasia
- dysarthria
- singing difficulty
- neck weakness

For treatment of Hemifacial spasm:
- facial weakness

For treatment of Focal dystonia:
- hand weakness and foot drop

Rare side effects have been reported but are not necessarily a result of the botulinum toxin. These include:
- nausea
- muscle soreness
- headaches
- light-headedness
- fever
- chills
- hypertension
- weakness
- difficulty breathing
- diarrhea
- abdominal pain

SPECIAL WARNING OF RISK TO FEMALES OF CHILDBEARING POTENTIAL

The effects of botulinum toxin type A on human babies are unknown, but could cause harm. For this reason it is necessary to:

- Use adequate birth control to avoid getting pregnant while receiving treatment.

- Inform me immediately if you get pregnant.

This treatment may cause an allergic reaction. Potentially, this reaction could be severe and life threatening.

As is true of all medications in medical treatment, there is always the possibility of a new or unexpected risk.

For the reasons stated above, if you have any worrisome symptoms please notify me immediately. My telephone number is _____ .

By signing this consent form, I acknowledge that I have read and understand this information and that Dr. _____ has explained the potential risks and benefits of this procedure to me. Additionally, there has been adequate time allowed for me to ask questions, and Dr. _____ has responded to my satisfaction.

_____

Signature of Patient   *Date*

_____

Signature of Witness   *Date*

When the patient is a minor or incompetent to give consent:

I, _____ hereby certify that I am

[relationship to patient] _____ of

[name of patient] _____

and am duly authorized to execute the foregoing.

_____

Signature   *Date*

_____

Signature of Witness   *Date*

ACETYLCHOLINE (ACh)—a neurotransmitter found in both the central and peripheral nervous system. The term, "cholinergic" refers to agents that have similar systemic actions of ACh. The acronym, SLUD, describes some cholinergic properties: **S**alivation, **L**acrimation, **U**rination, and **D**efecation.

ALPHA MOTOR NEURON—located in the ventral horn of the spinal cord, and innervates extrafusal skeletal muscle fibers. Alpha motor neurons, when improperly activated, may result in alpha rigidity due to disconnections between the cortex and one or more extrapyramidal tracts.

END-PLATE POTENTIAL (EPP)—a transient potential on the postjunctional muscle membrane due to ion currents (from sodium and potassium) caused from the binding of acetylcholine to the ionotropic (nicotinic) receptor on the muscle membrane. EPPs can be recorded using electromyography, and the precise location of the neuromuscular junction can be found. This information can help clinicians localize areas for BTX-A injections in some circumstances.

GLYCOLYSIS—process of breaking down glucose (a six-carbon sugar) into three-carbon structures (like pyruvate) creating high-energy intermediates (like ATP). Unlike oxidative phosphorylation, glycolysis does not require oxygen. Used by type II, fast-twitch muscle cells.

IONOTROPIC RECEPTOR—a membrane "pore" that opens directly upon ligand binding with a receptor allowing passage of ions. The nicotinic receptor, which binds acetylcholine, is a type of ionotropic receptor.

MEMBRANE-ASSOCIATED PROTEINS—many kinds of proteins are found in cell membranes, each with varying functions. One such protein,

SNAP-25, is degraded by BTX-A and thereby interferes with calcium-activated release of ACh from the nerve terminal. Other serotypes of the botulinum toxins (serotypes are designated A–F) act on different neuronal proteins, such as syntaxin or vesicle-associated membrane protein.

MUSCARINIC RECEPTOR—one of two types of acetylcholine receptors found in various smooth muscle and autonomic synapses throughout the body. Muscarinic receptors are blocked by atropine.

NEUROMUSCULAR JUNCTION—area between the nerve ending and receptor for acetylcholine. Usually found at the midpoint of each skeletal muscle fiber innervated. The collection of neuromuscular junctions makes up specific patterns, which can be simple or quite complex, in skeletal muscles.

NEUROTRANSMITTER—some experts define a neurotransmitter as a substance with the following properties: it is made within the neuron; activated by a calcium-dependent pathway; effects should be mimicked by exogenous application of the substance while blockade of receptors should abolish these effects; substance must be inactivated by metabolism or reuptake.

NICOTINIC RECEPTOR—one of two types of acetylcholine receptors found in various smooth muscle and autonomic synapses throughout the body. These receptors (nicotinic and muscarinic) are named because of their responses to plant alkaloids, muscarine and nicotine. Nicotinic receptors are found in skeletal muscle and at preganglionic sympathetic and parasympathetic synapses. Nicotinic receptors are blocked by curare.

NITRIC OXIDE (NO)—a highly permeable gas that acts like a neurotransmitter at synapses between inhibitory motor neurons and some smooth muscle cells. The enzyme NO synthase catalyzes the reaction arginine oxidation into citrulline and NO. NO synthase is stimulated by increased calcium ion inside an endothelial cell. The action of NO in smooth muscle is to relax the muscle.

NOCICEPTION—events in either the peripheral or central nervous system associated with the processing of nerve transmission elicited by tissue injury or the threat of tissue injury. Nociception differs from pain in that pain implies an unpleasant emotional response (a term reserved for humans, not animals). Unlike pain, nociception can occur under anesthesia. Thus, nociceptive events can be studied in anesthetized animals.

OXIDATIVE PHOSPHORYLATION—the biochemical pathway responsible for adding high-energy phosphate bonds to adenosine (creating adenosine triphosphate) and producing CO_2 while consuming molecular oxygen. (See TCA cycle in a chemistry text for a review of the chemistry.) Used by type I, slow-twitch muscle cells.

PERIPHERAL NERVOUS SYSTEM—everything outside of the central nervous system (brain and spinal cord). The peripheral nervous system is made up of the voluntary or somatic nervous system, which controls motor function, and the involuntary or autonomic nervous system, which controls visceral function (like blood pressure).

POSTGANGLIONIC—refers to the synapse after the ganglia in either the sympathetic or parasympathetic system. In the parasympathetic outflow, the postganglionic synapse is close to the target tissue. Acetylcholine acts on postganglionic muscarinic receptors in the parasympathetic system.

PREGANGLIONIC—refers to the synapse just prior to the first ganglia in the sympathetic or parasympathetic outflow. In the sympathetic system, the acetylcholine receptor is a nicotinic receptor.

SKELETAL MUSCLE—muscle attached to the body skeleton. Activation of skeletal muscle usually moves or stabilizes a joint.

SMOOTH MUSCLE—muscle that lines hollow organs or vessels. When smooth muscle contracts, it generally has a propulsive effect or a constrictive effect on its tissue.

SUBSTANCE P—a neuropeptide containing 11 amino acid residues with strong vasodilatory actions. It is a well-known modulator of nociceptive processes in both the central and peripheral nervous system. Release of substance P is blocked *in vitro* by botulinum toxins.